The Existential Crisis of Motherhood

Claire Arnold-Baker
Editor

The Existential Crisis of Motherhood

palgrave
macmillan

Editor
Claire Arnold-Baker
The New School of Psychotherapy and Counselling
London, UK

ISBN 978-3-030-56498-8 ISBN 978-3-030-56499-5 (eBook)
https://doi.org/10.1007/978-3-030-56499-5

Cover credit: SuperStock/Alamy Stock Photo

This Palgrave Macmillan imprint is published by the registered company Springer Nature Switzerland AG
The registered company address is: Gewerbestrasse 11, 6330 Cham, Switzerland

This book is dedicated to all mothers
But especially to my mother, Linda,
in loving memory.

Foreword

Before I became a mother, I used to think that books about motherhood were rather tedious and boring. They seemed to be written by and for women who thought that their lives could be fulfilled purely by being a mother. This appeared to me a rather self-limiting outlook, that offended my feminist instincts. I knew only too well that if my mother had chosen to be at home, as a housewife and mother, this was because she lived in another world, another era than I did. My parents had chosen for her to focus on raising the children and I felt deeply ambivalent about this insistence on the importance of motherly presence. It was obvious that my mother's considerable intelligence and her multiple talents had been wasted on raising my sister and me. She had so much spare capacity and was clearly frustrated, lavishing all her attention solely on her home and her family. This meant that we were all under far too much pressure to obey her demands and be eternally grateful for her care. It was oppressive and I suffocated. My teenage view was that children should be left to look after themselves. I craved freedom and independence and envied the latch key kids on our block. It seemed absurd to me that there were so many books telling women how to raise their children, when basically women should just leave their children alone to find their own way. When I came of age in the sixties, I wanted my horizon to be much wider than that and I swore I would never become the kind of mother who would hold her children to ransom in an over solicitous manner.

It soon became obvious to me how wrong I had been in my early dismissive condemnation. I struggled, in my twenties, to get pregnant, as my first marriage was infertile, and I deeply felt all the pain and dispossession of a woman who wants to procreate and is deprived of that immense privilege and pleasure. To make up for my lack I began looking after the children of friends and family and soon became aware of the overwhelming complexity and responsibility in getting this right. This period happily coincided with my studies in clinical psychology, which exposed me to many new theories about mothering, including psychoanalytic ones. But my previous philosophical background made me eager to reflect more deeply on these matters, challenging the assumptions people had about the way in which children experienced the world and in which mothers related to their babies. I became increasingly aware of the immensity of the transformation involved in bringing a child into the world and of the total absorption and responsibility it brought along with it.

It was an existential challenge that seemed vital to me in the process of becoming a whole person and therefore having a child became an important priority. My second marriage fortunately did bring this happy and fulfilling experience with it, together with the challenges of several pregnancies, natural and home childbirths, a miscarriage and the manifold ups and downs of the full ambiguity of motherhood. It felt as if I were finally being initiated into the rituals surrounding the true transition from child to adult and I prepared vigorously for the feat of giving birth to another human being. When it finally happened, in its full raw 24 hour struggle it left me with no doubt that it was one of the greatest physical challenges on earth. And though I had eagerly read as many books on pregnancy, birthing, childhood and motherhood as I could lay my hands on, I was in no way prepared for what was to come next. As soon as I was a mother, I felt unseen and unheard, unmet in my desire to make sense of the incredible transformations that were happening, to me, my body, my life, my own memories, my relationship to my parents, my relationship to my partner and husband, my relationship to my work and my career as a psychotherapist and academic. There simply was nothing and no one who had spoken to me honestly and directly about all the layers of this new and very wild adventure.

None of what I had read had touched upon the great hardship of seeing my pristine body burgeoning into new shapes and forms only to end up suffering an assault on its very survival. I felt forlorn carrying this new burden, on my own. Nobody really warned me of the many new and unsuspected problems visited upon me: the disturbed digestion and constipation, my decreased mobility, my low energy, my disrupted sleep patterns, my new unreasonably high expectations of myself in carrying on normally when everything was changed and in question. The books did not face up to the realities of my vital transformation, with its strange and eerie blossoming, that soon led to me taking up more space and needing bigger clothes, craving more self-indulgence, whilst yearning for more female or even maternal support, which at the same time I could not allow myself to ask for. I got slowly used to the feeling of my fertility with its weird sexual sensations of pressure in the groin, which weren't entirely pleasurable, the lack of periods, which were a boon and my altered relationship to all my natural functions. What to make of this changing body, with its more feminine profile, breasts enlarged twofold with their large brown nipples, that made me feel like mother nature herself had taken me over? What to make of the sudden spurt of that transparent liquid, preparing me for becoming the producer of plentiful mother's milk spurting forwards from this body that suddenly seemed to have a mind of its own? It all seemed so miraculous and overwhelming, but I was less inclined to intellectual discussion about it and learnt slowly but surely that the only way forward was to give in to it. The sheer mystery of the process of producing a baby without me having to know how to do this never ceased to amaze me. The enormous forces behind what was happening to me seemed beyond anything else I had ever known or experienced. How did my body know that it could harbour multiple spirits and create new life like this? How did it unfold the schedule of producing this other human being to perfection, as it did, despite my ignorance and self-doubt? How did it paint a brown stripe all down my abdomen from my pop-up belly button to my pelvis? How did it know to pace my labour and make me push with such vehemence during the process of birthing? I knew I had been taken over by another power that made me do all these things and I was in awe of the mystery, despite the fact I felt racked as my bones and my flesh were being stretched beyond what was tolerable.

And then that new phase took over, where I was immediately and irreversibly plunged into a love so deep and strong the moment, I laid eyes on my baby son and as I gently touched and smelled his tiny body, that it almost felt like another agony. How was it that I was being turned inside out a second time as this maternal instinct flooded over me? Now I was a plaything to a range of wild emotions that were to ensure that everything in a mental, social and spiritual sense was altered. I knew that I had never loved a human being with the fierce intensity with which I loved my baby. I felt like a wild animal in defending and protecting him. I would have done anything, including sacrificing my own existence, for his survival. I did not have to think or reflect on it. I would have put up with anything, including, as I had to, surviving on hardly any sleep for months on end.

But at the same time, I had met my emotional match. My child was very demanding and would not be fooled into anything. Appeasement was impossible. I felt continuously like a failure for not being able to get him to sleep or enable him to be awake in a more peaceful state. The worries were endless, the confrontation with my own limits and limitations was painful and humiliating. I questioned and doubted my ability like never before and never after. I often felt deficient and defective. It became obvious to me that those mothers who had not found books on mothering boring when they were young were far more capable than I was in looking after their offspring.

There was so much to learn and it was all so unstoppable and overwhelming, especially since I was the main breadwinner in my family and had, perhaps somewhat innocently and naively, committed to returning to work, almost immediately after the birth. The reality was that I had to earn a living and was self-employed. There were no family members to help out either. Our families both lived abroad, and we had very few contacts in the area we lived in. So, we were thrown in at the deep end without any real support. The existential crisis this created in my life went on for quite a while, before I became capable of absorbing all its lessons.

How I would have loved to have this book available to me at that time! How it would have helped me to know that many, nay most, other women feel the same way and that I was not exceptional in thinking myself ill prepared for motherhood and the ravages it brought to all aspects of my existence? With hindsight I travelled through months of depressive mood, and an anxiety so acute, that even if my baby slept occasionally, I often couldn't fall asleep myself, so worried was I that he would wake up again. I feared that I was not providing the right level of bonding and presence and had no idea that this particular child was especially challenging. For the longest time I blamed it all on myself and thought that his misery was due to my working as well as looking after him. When my husband began to take over some of the care, as our baby became less dependent on my nurturance, I began to blame my difficulties on the confusion that my child must feel in being parented by two different primary carers. Sometimes I also blamed it on my stress in heading up an academic department whilst being a mother in every sense of the word as well.

How I wish I had been given more reassurance, then. How I wish more mothers had shared their own worries and upsets, their self-doubts and their struggles. How I wish I had known from the outset that all my difficult moments and challenging transitions, my excruciating tiredness, my lack of confidence, my relentless guilt (towards baby, towards work), my yearning for safety and support were all just part and parcel of normal motherhood.

Perhaps the most important moment for me was when I brought my three-month-old baby with me to a four-day planning retreat of the teachers of one of the courses I was working on. Many of the other teachers were mature and experienced mothers and they handed my baby around the room for hours, cooing and dancing, and singing and laughing. It taught me the importance of community in child rearing and I never hesitated after that to bring my children with me, to work or wherever I went. It made everything a great deal easier and more casual as I gradually stopped fretting over whether I was doing the right thing and simply mucked in.

With hindsight I don't think the motherhood conundrum is about whether we get it right or wrong. It is about how quickly we allow ourselves to be destroyed and humbled by our new role, so that we can rebuild a new and much more flexible way of life and embrace a more easy-going and playful pattern. The longer we try to hold back the existential crisis of motherhood and the more time it will take before we allow ourselves to be moulded by the need to learn on the hoof, adjust and adapt to the needs of our children instead of trying to provide them with something that we think is preordained or written in stone, but is elusive and non-existent in reality.

Motherhood is to a large extent about letting go and giving in to nature. It is also about learning to respect the human need for cosiness and closeness, building an intimate world in which everything smells of goodness, home and safety. At the same time, it is about being confronted with every paradox under the sun: life and death are the very stuff of giving birth to a baby. Love and hate are having to be tamed as we experience each of these with great intensity in relation to this most adorable creature, who is a tyrant and will never obey our wishes and commands. We must allow ourselves to be pushed out of our previous shape and let ourselves be stretched to our limits, until we double our tolerance and expand our capacity for care, again and again, till it is sufficient. We deal with the magic of life and we get transported into great and lofty intuitions of a higher power, as soon as we see a new life suddenly emerging out of us, like a precious and unmerited gift. At the same time, we have to come to terms with our role in keeping up with the most basic earthly physical challenges, as our baby creates chaos and exposes us to all the human excretions we cannot speak about in polite company; the spit and the vomit, the faeces and the urine, the blood, the sweat, the curdled milk and the snot, every single day we are a mother.

This is what makes this book so exciting to me. For here we get to look at motherhood in the raw, as it is actually experienced by mothers. We also get to see it through the plural lenses of existential philosophy. We see the many different aspects of mothering that are not normally brought together. We are presented with the whole experience of this profoundly human endeavour and its inevitable effect of plunging us into existential crisis.

This book shows that motherhood is far from boring or trivial, the opposite of anodyne predictability. The chapters you are about to read are filled with the learning of women who have felt and reflected on motherhood deeply and who speak of it with a clear and fierce female intuition and sincerity. The message that emerges from it is passionate and instinctive and highly recommended to everyone who works in psychology, counselling or psychotherapy. These pages tell us things about being a mother that oblige and enable us to generate a new perspective. They witness of what is unspeakable and unmentionable and breathe fresh air over the age-old reality of bringing kids into this world, demonstrating how this affects and revolutionises our whole existence.

2019

Emmy van Deurzen
The New School of Psychotherapy and Counselling
London, UK

Preface

This book was conceived out of passion. A passion for women's voices to be heard and for experiences to be shared. For a private experience, which by its very nature is hidden, to be understood. Historically the maternal voice has been silenced either through science, reducing the mother to a biological process and instinct; or through religion, where the mother is seen as a vessel to receive and contain a baby which is given to them (Kristeva 2002). Neither discourse allows for the active part that women play in their maternal experience. Instead it is seen as something that either happens, or is done, to a woman. No understanding is elucidated by these two discourses on how this embodied experience impacts the totality of a woman's life. Through the systematic silencing of the maternal experience, women have been left isolated with messages which conflict with their actual experience. More recently numerous feminist authors and researchers have responded to this dearth of understanding with the aim of conceptualising or shifting the dominate maternal discourse. Many different theoretical viewpoints have been offered from which to examine the maternal experience, and these have included psychological, feminist, psychoanalytical, anthropological or sociological perspectives. This book offers a new existential perspective that will join, and add to, these increasingly emphatic voices.

A shift has been occurring, however, within the medical field, where a greater understanding of the complexity of the mother's experience is now being acknowledged. This has been demonstrated for example by the creation of the Maternal Mental Health Alliance, whose aim is to create a network of maternal mental health support across the UK during pregnancy and the first year of birth. A number of other organisations have also emerged such as MumsAid, Make Birth Better and the Birth Trauma Association. All of which recognise the need for attending to the mental health of women during pregnancy and postnatally. But it takes time for these changing discourses to filter through to the general population. In the meantime, women are often left to grapple with making sense of their experiences on their own.

There is also a greater understanding of the nuances of the maternal experience and the diverse ways in which women can be mothers; and of the multitude ways in which women can be affected. No longer is it assumed that all mothers who struggle postnatally are suffering from postnatal depression (PND). In fact, mothers who struggle may be depressed, or they may find motherhood an anxiety inducing experience and suffer from postnatal anxiety (PNA), or they may be facing an experience of birth trauma, which has led to PTSD. In extreme cases, mothers may also experience postpartum psychosis. While it is useful to use these diagnostic labels as they confer a certain meaning and understanding and provide a language with which we can communicate and focus support; there is a danger that it continues to medicalise the maternal experience, keeping it confined within a biological and scientific perspective. This focus on the struggles that women experience also overshadows the fact that pregnancy, birth and motherhood can also be positive experiences for women, as Hill has stressed in her book *The Positive Birth Book* (2017). A medical perspective has certainly improved mortality rates for mothers and babies, but it comes at a cost. That is not to say that this cost is not worth taking but there may be ways in which the two can coexist to ensure that the mother has the best experience possible.

This book, therefore, aims to offer an alternative perspective, grounded in the experiential accounts of women and understood through a philosophical lens. Philosophy can offer a new way in which we can understand motherhood as part of our human experience. Existential philosophers (e.g. Sartre 1943; Heidegger 1962; Kierkegaard 1844) in particular have striven towards elucidating the fundamental structures of human experience. They were interested in uncovering the ontological aspects that we all share as human beings; the fundamentals that we all struggle with and which form the existential ground on which we stand. The majority of these writers and thinkers were, however, men and although they were concerned with disclosing the universal aspects of human existence, it allowed for a male-dominated discourse. There were exceptions of course, the most notable being Simone De Beauvoir and her book *The Second Sex*. De Beauvoir's feminist position examined the roles and responsibilities that are inherent in being a woman and a mother, although De Beauvoir was never a mother herself. Writing in 1949, she argued that societal ideas confine the woman in her role of mother, making it difficult for women to raise themselves above these responsibilities and confirm themselves as individuals. Whilst much has changed for women since the time de Beauvoir was writing, they are still struggling with aspects of this today. These themes have been taken up more recently by Butterfield (2010) who stated that women are always more than their maternal identity due to their fundamental freedom. Mothers occupy a unique position in that they are intensely bound to another, their child, and yet at the same time they are free. Motherhood is therefore ambiguous, argues Butterfield, mothers are both individual and social and both free and determined; it is up to each mother to choose how she will live that identity.

This tension, that is created for women when they become mothers, has also been explored by Badinter (2010) a French philosopher, who argues that there are no philosophical distinctions between men and women, we are all human and that being defined as 'mother' separates women from men. Other authors have also explored the notion that the mother's role is socially constructed rather than innately given (Miller 2005). Whilst it is clear that either gender can take care of and be responsible for a new-born child, a woman's biology usually designates the role of 'mother'. This is a notion that has been challenged by Trans fathers and the discourse around gender fluidity. Witt (2020) argues that we should think about gender in terms of social norms rather than gender kinds. She proposes a *gender uniessentialism*, which highlights how social roles are created along gender norms. This suggests that a person's gender would presuppose a normative response in a social situation, where a woman would be expected to act in one way and a man in another. In patriarchal societies, Witt (2020) observes, women are disadvantaged 'because social roles are gendered in an asymmetrical fashion, in a manner that is oppressive to women'. This raises interesting questions about the concept of 'mother' but also highlights how social norms exist to maintain the status quo in a society. As Witt and others have noted, gender norms create a power imbalance between men and women but they also have the effect of maintaining pro-natal societies. Brown (2019) argues that economies are constructed in such a way that they need women to reproduce to ensure a continued supply of workers and consumers and so gender norms are created to support this. Norms such as babies need mothers, the maternal instinct, and that motherhood and childbirth are 'natural', all create expectations for mothers and a normative discourse into which women are thrown. This can be confusing for mothers as they move from a discourse where they are needed and valued in the workforce to one where they are essential to the home and their baby. It is little wonder that women often struggle with the work-home balance. It is because they are caught up in two opposing normative positions that women take in society.

The tension caused around gender and societal roles has provoked much discussion amongst feminist thinkers and writers. From a philosophical perspective there are no ontological differences between the genders, we all face the same limits to our existence, we all have to confront our freedom, choice and responsibilities and to face our facticity. Yet there is also something inherently unique about the maternal experience. It may be difficult to claim that maternity is an ontological phenomenon in its own right, as it is not experienced by everyone, but maternity does have the effect that existence is experienced in a unique way. This is not to say that all women will experience being a mother in the same way as there are many diverse ways in which women can be mothers, but there are some shared ontological features of motherhood which all women experience as will be shown throughout this book.

In recent years, female philosophers in the UK have turned their attention towards birth and being born. There has been renewed interest recently in Arendt's (2018) concept of *natality*, the act of being born. Stone (2019), whose recently published book, *Being Born: Birth and Philosophy*, stresses the equal importance of natality and mortality to a person's existence. Whereas mortality throws the end of our existence into sharp relief conveying a sense of anxiety to our lives, natality also impacts how we live our lives. Both concern our non-existence, but natality refers to our non-existence before we were born and therefore determines our experience of *thrownness* (Heidegger 1962). Stone posits that natality highlights the relational aspects of human existence, which she states as being dependency, relationality, situatedness and embeddedness. Our natality shows how vulnerable human beings are at birth and how much our survival depends on others. But that we are always in a certain context, situated in the world in a particular time and place and embedded into a certain society. Human existence, therefore, is bound by both our natality and mortality. Natality brings into focus our understanding of our own birth and the impact that has on our life, our relationships and our sense of non-being. According to Rank (2014), our own birth leaves us with feelings of anxiety because the birth is experienced as traumatic. Whilst the focus of natality is on how being born impacts our human existence, the experience of the birthing mother has not, however, been totally neglected by philosophers. Staehler (2016, 2017, 2018) has phenomenologically explored aspects of the embodied experience of pregnancy and birth from an existential and philosophical perspective. This interest in a philosophical or spiritual dimension to the experience of birth has also been found in the midwifery field. Crowther and Hall's (2018) edited book *Spirituality and Childbirth: Meaning and Care at the Start of Life* brings together recent research in this area from an existential or philosophical perspective. It is encouraging to see how a phenomenological exploration of pregnancy and birth can provide much insight into a woman's experience and this current book aims to do the same for motherhood.

Whilst existential philosophy has largely ignored the female experience, the same is also true of the field of existential therapy. Again, this field has been characterised by its male dominance despite the approach having been firmly established in the UK, by Emmy van Deurzen in 1982 (du Plock and Tantam 2019), when she set up the first training in existential therapy. Although maternity has mainly been underrepresented as an area of concern amongst existential therapists, there have been a small number of authors who have addressed this area. A leading figure is Naomi Stadlen, whose two books '*What Mothers Do*' (2005) and '*How Mothers Love*' (2011) provide a phenomenological description of the experience of early motherhood. Other authors have included Deurzen (1998, 2002 and 2009) who has written about her own experience of being a mother as well as case studies about her work with postnatal mothers and Goldenberg (1997) and Goldenberg and Tikvah (2000) who explored infertility from an existential perspective. Arnold-Baker and Donaghy (2005) elucidated the existential dimensions of procreation, which developed out of their masters' research into the transition to motherhood. Donaghy, a former NSPC student and Founder of MumsAid, focussed her research (2001) on exploring whether postnatal depression could be viewed as an existential crisis, whereas Arnold-Baker (2000) examined how the transition to motherhood evoked a crisis of the self, as well as a life crisis, for first-time mothers.

Therefore, the aim of this book is threefold; to provide experiential accounts of motherhood and in particular those early stages of being a mother; to offer a philosophical understanding of maternity and finally to demonstrate how an understanding of existential themes and ontological structures can be helpful when working with mothers therapeutically. Above all, this book aims to challenge the dominant discourses on maternity and to offer a female voice to counter those many male voices in the field of philosophy and existential therapy.

The passion for this book emerged from the passion of each of the contributors, for which I am grateful, to investigate and think deeply about an area of motherhood that was meaningful to each of us. Together we have tried to make sense of something that is difficult to understand, and to stand firmly in the face of uncertainty. What this book offers is a new perspective, by uncovering more questions than it is able to answer, it is hoped that it will engage the reader in a deep reflection of the maternal experience and what that also means for our human existence.

This book would not have been possible without the many women who took part in the various pieces of research, attended therapy sessions at MumsAid (informing Chapter 8) or joined weekly discussion groups for mothers in North London (informing Chapter 5); their voices have informed the proceeding chapters. The mothers gave up their time freely, in order that by sharing their experiences they can help other women understand the phenomenon of motherhood and all that it entails. Gaining a collective description of the motherhood experience that women will be able to recognise and feel connected to and ease their feelings of isolation.

I would also like to thank all the other research supervisors at the New School of Psychotherapy and Counselling (NSPC) who, along with myself, were involved in the various pieces of research for their interest, input and support; Prof. Emmy van Deurzen, Dr. Claire Asherson Bartram, Dr. Patricia Bonnici, Prof. Simon Du Plock, Dr. Jacqui Farrants, Dr. Charlotte Harkness, Dr. Rosemary Lodge, Dr. Chloe Paidousis-Mitchell and Naomi Stadlen. Finally, I would like to thank Sasha van Deurzen-Smith for the valuable conversations we had around gender fluidity.

London, UK Claire Arnold-Baker

References

Arendt, H. (2018). *The Human Condition* (2nd ed.). Chicago: University of Chicago Press (1958).

Arnold-Baker, C. (2000). *Life Crisis or Crisis of the Self?: An Existential View of Motherhood* (Unpublished MA Dissertation). Sheffield: NSPC and University of Sheffield.

Arnold-Baker, C., & Donaghy, M. (2005). Procreation. In E. van Deurzen & C. Arnold-Baker (Eds.), *Existential Perspectives on Human Issues*. London: Palgrave Macmillan.

Badinter, E. (2010). *The Conflict: How Modern Motherhood Undermines the Status of Women* (Trans. A. Hunter). New York: Metropolitan Books.

Brown, J. (2019). *Birth Strike: The Hidden Fight Over Women's Work.* Michigan: PM Press.

Butterfield, E. (2010). 'Days and Nights of a New Mother': Existentialism in the Nursery. In S. Linott (Ed.), *Motherhood: Philosophy for Everyone*. West Sussex: Wiley-Blackwell.

Crowther, S., & Hall, J. (Eds.). (2018). *Spirituality and Childbirth: Meaning and Care at the Start of Life*. Abingdon: Routledge.

De Beauvoir, S. (1997). *The Second Sex*. London: Vintage.

Deurzen, E. van (1998). *Paradox and Passion in Psychotherapy: An Existential Approach to Therapy and Counselling*. Chichester: Wiley.

Deurzen, E. van (2002). *Existential Counselling and Psychotherapy in Practice* (2nd ed.). London: Sage.

Deurzen, E. van (2009). *Psychotherapy and the Quest for Happiness.* London: Sage.

Donaghy, M. (2001). *Postnatal Depression: An Existential Crisis* (Unpublished MA Dissertation). Sheffield: NSPC and University of Sheffield.

Du Plock, S., & Tantam, D. (2019). History of Existential-Phenomenological Therapy. In E. van Deurzen et al. (Eds.), *The Wiley World Handbook of Existential Therapy*. Chichester: Wiley Blackwell.

Goldenberg, H. (1997). Who Am I If I Am Not a Mother. In S. Du Plock (Ed.), *Case Studies from an Existential Perspective.* Chichester: Wiley.

Goldenberg, H., & Tikvah, S. E. (2000). Living Infertility. In S. Rothschild & S. Sheridan (Eds.), *Taking Up the Timbrel*. London: SCM Press.

Heidegger, M. (1962). *Being and Time.* (Trans. J. Macquarrie & E. S. Robinson). Malden, MA, and Oxford: Blackwell (1927).

Hill, M. (2017). *The Positive Birth Book.* London: Printer and Martin.

Kierkegaard, S. (1844). *The Concept of Anxiety* (Trans. R. Thomte). Princeton, NJ: Princeton University Press (1980).

Kristeva, J. (2002). Maternity, Feminism and Female Sexuality. In K. Oliver (Ed.). *The Portable Kristeva.* New York: Columbia University Press.

Miller, T. (2005). *Making Sense of Motherhood: A Narrative Approach.* Cambridge: Cambridge University Press.

Rank, O. (2014). *The Trauma of Birth.* London: Routledge.

Sartre, J. P. (1943). *Being and Nothingness.* London: Routledge.

Stadlen, N. (2005). *What Mothers Do: Especially When It Looks Like Nothing.* London: Piatkus.

Stadlen, N. (2011). *How Mothers Love and How Relationships Are Born.* London: Piatkus.

Staehler, T. (2016). Passivity, Being-With and Being-There: Care During Birth. *Medicine, Health Care and Philosophy: A European Journal, 19*(3), 371–279.

Staehler, T. (2017). Who's Afraid of Birth? Exploring Mundane and Existential Affects with Heidegger. *Janus Head, 16*(1).

Staehler, T. (2018). Pregnant Embodiment as World Transformation. In A. Cimino & C. Leijenhorst (Eds.), Phenomenology and Experience: New Perspectives. *Studies in Contemporary Phenomenology*, 18.

Stone, A. (2019). *Being Born: Birth and Philosophy*. Oxford: Oxford University Press.

Witt, C. (2020). Gender Essences. Available from: https://aeon.co/essays/would-you-be-the-same-person-if-you-were-a-different-gender. Accessed June 2020.

Contents

Notes on Contributors

Claire Arnold-Baker is a UKCP reg existential psychotherapist and HCPC reg counselling psychologist who specialises in working with mothers. Claire is also Academic Manager at the New School of Psychotherapy and Counselling where she is also Course Leader for the DCPsych programme. She is a senior lecturer, clinical and research supervisor and author, having co-edited *Existential Perspectives on Human Issues* (2005) with Emmy van Deurzen with whom she also co-authored *Existential Therapy: Distinctive Features* (2018). Claire is passionate about maternal mental health and a strong advocate for improving and supporting women's maternal experience. www.mothertime.co.uk.

Josephine Coates-Davies is a UKCP registered existential psychotherapist and coach, and a lecturer at the New School of Psychotherapy and Counselling. She specialises in helping people to access and express their creative energy and holds a belief that creativity is an intrinsic aspect of being human, not just something for the privileged few. She has a particular interest in the social aspects of gender and identity, and the relationship between the personal and the political. She is currently on sabbatical from client work in order to focus on her career as an improvising musician and composer. www.josephinedavies.co.uk.

Miriam Donaghy, FRSA is a UKCP registered psychotherapist with 20 years' experience of specialising in perinatal mental health. She is the founder and Chief Executive of MumsAid, a multi, award-winning charity that supports maternal mental health. Prior to founding MumsAid, Miriam managed parenting projects for Greenwich Mind and the Tavistock (TCCR), developing innovative services for new mothers and training for frontline professionals. She also developed the Baby and Me programme for mothers with complex needs. Miriam has published articles in several magazines and journals and has won two awards for her 'Significant Contribution by an Individual' in developing Perinatal Mental Health services.

Aoife Gaffney has been working as an Art Psychotherapist and Cognitive Behavioural Therapist for the past eleven years. In later years, her training has included Existential Psychology (NSPC & Middlesex University). Aoife has been a lecturer for eleven years in the area of Counselling, Cognitive Behavioural Therapy and Existential Counselling. She is currently a lecturer and supervisor in the Psychology Department of Dublin Business School in Ireland. Her academic, research and clinical training inspired her use of Creative Existential Therapy Practices, and she is an advocate for using existential creative methods with mothers as a form of therapeutic reflection. She is affiliated with the BPS, APCP and BABCP.

Victoria Garland is a counselling psychologist and an existential psychotherapist. Victoria works as a Deputy Course Leader for the DCPsych programme at New School of Psychotherapy and Counselling (NSPC); she is a clinical supervisor, researcher supervisor and a lecturer. Also, Victoria is one of the founders and a trustee of a charity called 'Cocoon Family Support', that is a London-based charity supporting those affected by ante- and postnatal depression, and those struggling to deal with difficult emotions before and after birth. 'Cocoon Family Support' offer a range of services including, guided peer support groups, one-to-one counselling, workshops and many more.

Susan Harris is from the UK and affiliated with UKCP as a registered existential psychotherapist. She completed her Doctoral research in traumatic bereavement at the New School of Psychotherapy and Counselling, specialising in trauma and bereavement in adults. She currently works in a primary care mental health support service in the NHS. Prior to training as an existential psychotherapist she worked in education and teaching in Japan, and holds an MSc in Applied Linguistics, and an MSc in Psychotherapy Studies.

Naomi Magnus is a UKCP and BACP registered existential psychotherapist, based in London, England. She has 20 years' experience in youth work, training youth leaders and supporting young people with their emotional and mental well-being. Naomi has worked in a variety of counselling settings and has travelled extensively, working with non-profit community and human rights organisations. Since becoming a mother in 2016 Naomi has become passionate about supporting women at each phase of their motherhood journey. Naomi currently works in private practice in North London and has 2 young children who are keeping her occupied.

Julie McCarthy is an Existential-Phenomenological Counselling Psychologist who completed her training at Regent's College and the New School of Psychotherapy and Counselling in London. She is a highly specialist trauma therapist for the Government of Jersey working with complex PTSD, personality disorders and dissociative disorders. She is also an online tutor and academic supervisor at the New School of Psychotherapy and Counselling in London and a clinical supervisor in private practice. She is a mother of three and lives on the Island of Jersey in the Channel Islands.

Jennifer Ofori UKCP reg, (MBACP) is a qualified and fully accredited counselling psychotherapist who has gained experience working in private, voluntary educational and public sectors—which includes her work: for an IAPT/NHS service offering counselling to clients on a short-term basis based in London. As a registered counselling psychotherapist, she currently works in private practice with adults and members of the younger generation. Jennifer completed her doctoral research at the New School of Psychotherapy and Counselling (NSPC), which explored the experiences of first time British mothers of second-generateon Ghanaian descent.

Farasat Sadia has a Masters in Psychology and Doctorate in Counselling Psychology & Psychotherapy. She is a graduate member of the BPS and an accredited member of UKCP. Farasat is an existential psychotherapist with experience of working in the NHS, education, private and third sector settings. She is currently working as a Psychotherapist at the University of Cambridge Counselling Services looking after students suffering from mental health & lifestyle issues. She strongly leans towards an existential phenomenological approach in both research and practice. Her aim is to enable her clients to face the anxieties of life head on and to embrace the freedom of choice everyone possesses.

Romy Shulman is an existential psychotherapist in London, England and is a member of the BPS. She has an M.Sc. in Psychological Counselling and a Doctorate in Counselling Psychology. She has over 12 years' experience working in the mental health field in both the NHS and the charity sector. Her current specialism is in counselling related to infertility. She is the clinical manager at Chana, a charity supporting couples facing infertility, birth trauma and perinatal mental health difficulties. Romy's Doctoral research explored the experience of mothering a very premature infant in the first year after hospital discharge.

Elizabeth Simmons is an Existential Counselling Psychologist who completed her doctoral training with the New School of Psychotherapy and Counselling. For her thesis, she combined her interest in philosophical approaches to living with uncertainty with a desire to amplify the voices of new mothers. She chose a narrative approach, influenced by her pre-psychology background as an English Literature graduate and media professional. She has since worked clinically with survivors of abuse, refugees, and for Rochdale and District Mind. She now runs a

Manchester-based consultancy, Horizon Psychological Services, and is a mother of two.

Naomi Stadlen may have been the first to have studied existentialism at a British university. In 1963, the University of Sussex offered an existential course, and only she signed up. Now a mother and grandmother, she is an existential psychotherapist in London; teaches at the New School of Psychotherapy and Counselling; and runs Mothers Talking, a weekly discussion group for mothers. Her three books are: *What Mothers Do—Especially When It Looks Like Nothing* (2004); *How Mothers Love—and How Relationships are Born* (2011); and *What Mothers Learn—Without Being Taught* (2020). www.naomistadlen.com.

List of Figures

List of Tables

Part I

Existential Crisis: The Philosophical Tensions of Being a Mother

1

Introduction: The Existential Crisis of Motherhood

Claire Arnold-Baker

The Existential Crisis of Motherhood

Crisis is not usually a word associated with motherhood. It is most often described or thought of as a joyful and happy event, that is wanted and expected and therein lies the paradox of motherhood. It evokes powerful emotional responses which are often contradictory. Can an experience be both joyful and shocking? Induce intense love but also frustration? Evoke deep feelings of guilt but also pride. It is this ambiguity surrounding the experience of motherhood which has also led to the plethora of research and literature in this area. Research which aims to capture the essence of an experience which feels on the one hand ethereal and other worldly but at the same time is corporeal and grounded.

The word crisis usually conjures up an image of great emotional turmoil and distress; a time of extreme trouble or danger (Collins Dictionary 1993). But viewing motherhood in this way is to look at only

C. Arnold-Baker (✉)
The New School of Psychotherapy and Counselling, London, UK
e-mail: claire@nspc.org.uk

C. Arnold-Baker (ed.), *The Existential Crisis of Motherhood*,
https://doi.org/10.1007/978-3-030-56499-5_1

one side of the equation. Monk (2013) warns that making motherhood a crisis accounts for its medicalisation and the resultant need for intervention. Whilst this may be the experience of those mothers who have experienced birth trauma, for example, it isn't the experience of all mothers. Yet the transition to motherhood is a significant period of time for all mothers. It's complexity, therefore, is due to there being myriad experiences for women, where each mother's journey is unique.

There are, however, other types of crisis, which are not so traumatic in that an individual would feel in danger, but which serve to turn our lives upside down. These periods of crisis are momentous times in one's life which cause us to stop and think again. They create periods of unsettledness that can lead to a questioning or re-evaluation of our lives. Typically, they occur at major life transitions, such as adolescence, midlife or retirement. But they can also arise at other crisis points in our lives, such as redundancy, bereavement or the loss of a relationship.

All of these times of crisis involve a period in which the person's life changes, often suddenly and in unexpected ways. The normal patterns or routines of life are disrupted, either by events, change in circumstances or changes to the individual's relationship to themselves or other people. Times of crisis have been described as 'everything is turned upside down' (Deurzen 2009: 107), or as a 'disruption of the normal course of life' (Jacobsen 2006: 42) or as 'something extraordinary and personally decisive' (Bollnow 1959 cited Jacobsen 2006: 42). As Deurzen states, 'crises may also occur in ordinary situations or even events that would seem apparently happy, such as pregnancy or birth' (Deurzen 2009). The changes that occur during a crisis often lead to a re-examination of an individual's life, when they rethink their values and beliefs and how they see themselves and their lives. These periods are often quite difficult and intense. It takes time for an individual to make sense of what has happened to them and to begin to see their lives in new ways.

Maternity as Life Crisis

In Jacobsen's (2006) exploration of the phenomenon of life crisis, he elucidates three dimensions of a crisis: crisis as adversity, crisis as loss and crisis as an opening of existence. The adversity that Jacobsen refers to describes what one would normally associate with crisis; an adverse event or situation that must be overcome. These events are often out of our control and are subject to chance. They involve 'boundary situations' (Jaspers 1951), the limits to our existence to which individuals must decide how they respond, or what attitude they choose to take towards the challenges they represent (Frankl 1964). As Jacobsen (2006) states, these crises cannot be changed and therefore need to be accepted as the individual's existential ground.

Crisis can also involve a loss, this can be a loss of something material or relational, i.e. the loss of a person due to bereavement or the loss of a job or a home, but it also concerns an individual's loss of meaning or a loss to their worldview. Likewise, this sense of loss may concern a person's sense of themselves, where their values and beliefs are challenged by events or situations out of their control.

When motherhood is viewed through this lens the loss is not initially apparent. Mothers gain a new baby and a new way of life. Yet mothers also lose a sense of the 'old me' and feel that life will never be the same again. The paradox of motherhood is that with gains there are also losses too, you cannot have one without the other—they are two sides of the same coin. The mother's meaning in life changes on the birth of her baby (Arnold-Baker 2015; Prinds et al. 2013); her priorities change but there are also changes in her views about herself and her life. Although there is often a gap after the birth before mothers are able to assimilate and make sense of their new ways of being. It is this aspect of loss that Jacobsen refers to as a 'loss of the unfolding of life'. Although for motherhood this rupture is a welcomed one, it is still a rupture in a woman's existence. A rupture which is expected but also sudden—in the moment of birth everything changes.

Motherhood, therefore, is a crisis moment for women; one which can be experienced as either an adversity, a loss or an unfolding of existence. Raphael (1975) conceptualised the *rite de* passage of 'mother-becoming' as *Matrescence* and likens it to adolescence, in terms of the many changes; physical, emotional and hormonal that occur. If adolescence is seen as a crisis point in a person's life, then so too must motherhood.

In fact, anthropological cross-cultural studies have shown that the physiological experiences of childbirth are 'almost universally treated as a traumatic life crisis event' (Kruckman 1992: 139). Many cultures mark this period in a ritualised or structured way, which indicates a transition in social roles and gives the new mother time to recuperate and for her needs and tasks to be taken care of. This integration phase which follows what is seen as a major life transition helps mothers to incorporate and become absorbed into their new social state (Van Gennep 2004). Yet in Western Society there is little social support for new mothers and 'no formal social structuring of the puerperium[1] once the mother has returned home' (Kruckman 1992: 138) and so women are left to overcome this traumatic life crisis, and work things out for themselves, with little or no support.

Existential Crisis

The crisis of motherhood takes on a new perspective when we consider the Greek origins of the word, *Krisis*—meaning to decide or to choose. From this viewpoint, motherhood becomes a time when women are expected to make many decisions and choices not only for their newborns but also for themselves as well. Everything must be chosen, and women become aware of the enormity of these choices. This is brought to the fore because a woman's life has changed totally and forever when she has a baby. It is a transformation which mothers are never fully able to prepare for: as Dani explains 'So as much as you can be prepared, I don't know if anything quite prepares you for the experience' (Arnold-Baker 2015: 134). Motherhood also becomes a time when women are confronted with the basic tenets of existence: of life and death; and of the complex interaction between choice, freedom and responsibility (Arnold-Baker and Donaghy 2005; Arnold-Baker 2015). This focus, that occurs in early motherhood, sheds light on how we understand and experience

[1]**Puerperium:** The time immediately after the delivery of a baby. (In Latin a "puerpera" is a woman in childbirth since "puer" means child and "parere" means to give birth.) (MedicineNet.com, 2003).

our existence in all its richness. Which means that we need to treat the crisis of motherhood as an existential one.

An existential crisis is quite distinct from the usual definition of crisis—although all types of crisis might also lead to an existential crisis. More specifically an existential crisis occurs when we stop to consider our existence in its entirety. When we question our life, our values and beliefs and the meaning and purpose we give to our lives. As with the Greek *Krisis*, an existential crisis requires us to make a decision about our existence. We experience an existential crisis when we are confronted with the unpredictable nature of our lives. When we come to realise that the expectations we have of life are also subject to chance. Jaspers (1951) describes these as the limitations of our existence or boundary situations, these unknown aspects of existence which come into play despite our best intentions. This is most keenly seen during the birth process where mothers, having thought about and made their birth plans, are confronted with the unpredictable nature of birth. In those moments, mothers become aware of the many other possibilities that are now opening up for them and which they had not previously considered or were even able to grasp beforehand. The birth process, and therefore motherhood, creates a situation of *thrownness* for mothers; a term Heidegger (1962) used to denote the arbitrary and unfathomable nature of existence. He believed that we are always *thrown* into a world that we did not choose. Whilst this is certainly true for the new-born baby, it is also true for the mother. The mother becomes aware that her sense of her life has changed immeasurably, that she is subject to chance and that there are elements of her life that she cannot choose or control. A known world has been replaced by an unknown one. This is when our 'everyday familiarity collapses' (Heidegger 1962: 189) and we move 'into the existential "mode" of the "not-at-home"' (ibid.: 189). The feeling of 'not-at-home' or *umheimlich* describes, according to Heidegger, the uncanny nature of existence. We move from being absorbed by the world, to seeing the world as it really is. Although this unfamiliarity or feeling of being 'not-at-home' are anxiety provoking they also highlight the mother's freedom and therefore her ability to choose. It is ironic that at a time when women are creating a sense of 'home' for themselves which comes with the birth of their baby, they also feel the most 'not-at-home' in their lives. Mothers have described this as entering the *unknown*, an aspect that is unfamiliar to them and where they feel there is no solid ground beneath their feet (Arnold-Baker 2015). This is another paradoxical tension for mothers to face. Yet it is through feeling 'not-at-home' that mothers are able to create this new family environment, and in time, a sense of themselves as mothers. The struggle that comes with facing these tensions provides them with the energy to create and overcome and to break free of old ways of living.

Being aware that there are other possibilities than were previously evident, highlights a person's choice which in turn reveals their personal freedom and ultimately their responsibility. Freedom, choice and responsibility are inextricably linked and as soon as we become aware that we have the freedom to choose then our responsibility for those choices becomes apparent and this in turn causes us to feel anxiety. Sartre sums this up when he says that 'man is condemned to be free' (Sartre 1943: 553), that the price of freedom is responsibility because if we are free to choose then we are responsible for those choices. New mothers are very aware of this and their new responsibility towards their babies, as they recognise the impact their choices can have on their babies' lives. Mothers experience this existential given in a practical sense, but it is a burden; as they have no way of knowing if the choices that they make are going to be good ones.

Kierkegaard was notable in stating that our human predicament meant that we had to live our lives forward, but we could only understand them backwards (Kierkegaard 1844). It is only in hindsight that we can know how our choices will play out; effectively we are living our lives blind to the future but having to choose anyway. Kierkegaard stated that this is the nature of our human existence, that we have to choose and to suffer from our choices. This causes us to experience anxiety or *angst* as he termed it. Existential anxiety, or *angst*, is also experienced when we become aware of our freedom and the inevitable responsibility that it brings (Sartre 1943). Both these experiences of *angst* arise from the awareness of our human condition which becomes so apparent during the birth and early motherhood. Further existential anxiety arises from the awareness that we are limited in time, we are Being-towards-death, and our future is unknown to us (Heidegger 1962). Freedom, choice, responsibility and temporality are essential tenets of existential thought which seek to describe the fundamental elements of our human existence.

When motherhood is examined from an existential perspective, it becomes clear that mothers experience, in varying degrees, an existential crisis. The mothers' life is totally transformed by the birth of her baby. The birth brings forth an awareness of death, both her own death, and that of her baby's. The vulnerability of the baby highlights the mother's responsibility to herself and the responsibility she now has towards her baby (Arnold-Baker 2015; Garland 2019). The mother has to choose, or decide, many things in those early days, months and years and her choices will have a huge impact on her baby and its life, yet, there is no way for the mother to know the consequences of these choices. This all compounds in making mothers rethink and re-evaluate their lives, and themselves, as they strive to discover what is important for them. Mothers often talk about shifting priorities and finding different aspects meaningful after the birth of their babies (Prinds et al. 2013; Arnold-Baker 2015). Mothers become tuned into existence in a new way. They become aware of the basic tenets of existence, of life and death, and of their freedom and responsibility. Mothers will often try to control their experience through reading books and talking to others to alleviate the existential anxiety they experience but will soon have to face the reality that the future is unknown and uncontrollable. All they can control are the choices that they make at that point in time and to be open to the new possibilities that open up to them. Arnold-Baker argued that 'If the mother's intentions are good, then she will make the best possible choice that she can in that moment, based on the situation she finds herself in.' (Arnold-Baker 2019: 9) but also grounded in what she currently knows about herself, her baby and the world.

Existential Re-Birth

The complexity of motherhood has been shown to involve changes on all four dimensions of existence, in the physical, social, personal and spiritual realms (Arnold-Baker 2015). This research confirms the uncanny nature of motherhood, that there is no dimension in their lives in which mothers feel settled and secure or 'at-home'. Stern and his wife, Nadia Bruschweiler-Stern's (1998) research found that a 'mother has to be born psychologically as much as her baby is born physically. What a woman gives birth to in her mind is not a new human being, but a new identity: the sense of being a mother' (Stern and Bruschweiler-Stern 1998: 3). They believed that mothers need to undergo a psychological transition in order to allow their new motherhood identities to develop. This psychological transition is also an embodied one which begins in pregnancy, where the woman's changing body allows mothers to relinquish their previous sense of self and to enable a new sense of being a mother to grow (Stern and Bruschweiler-Stern 1998; McCarthy 2015).

The mother, however, is not only born psychologically, motherhood is also a time of 'existential re-birth' (Deurzen 2009). Deurzen describes how times of crisis have a transformational effect on people. That the process of overcoming adversity or life's difficulties often leads to a transformation or development in the individual. Deurzen highlights this by drawing on images such as the phoenix rising from the ashes. The existential crisis of motherhood is one such transformative process. Mothers face a new awareness of the existential and ontological structures of their existence, as well as the accompanying changes to their sense of self, their relationships with others and the new world that they now find themselves in. All these aspects contribute to the existential re-birth of mothers. Mothers are re-born existentially when they are confronted with the reality of their existence. A window of awareness opens up to them in those early months of motherhood which form part of the existential crisis that they experience, and this inevitably leads to a transformation as mothers renegotiate this new life.

Creating Existential Space

A significant element of the transformation that mothers undertake is their ability to create space in their life for their babies. This begins during pregnancy when the mother creates space for her baby in a physical and embodied way; her body changing to accommodate the growing foetus. But the mother must also create psychological and emotional space for the baby too and Stadlen notes that this entails a 'momentous inner shift' (Stadlen 2005: 185–186). It changes the mother profoundly and is a complicated process which requires the mother to no longer think 'of herself as a self-contained "I"' (ibid.: 118). Stadlen believes that creating this psychological space develops out of the mother's relationship with her baby. Relating to a baby requires a slower pace of life and as part of this slowing down process mothers become more aware of their babies but also everything else around them (ibid.: 190). Through this awareness, the mother opens herself up and it is this openness, receptivity and attentiveness that enables the mother to create a space within herself for her baby. Stadlen calls this *heartroom*, drawing on Kierkegaard's (1962) notion of up-building: 'if a mother opens up real heartroom for her child, it does not seem possible to fold it away again' (Stadlen 2011: 18). This *heartroom* or openness allows the possibility for the mother to gain an understanding of her baby and the baby's needs and desires which leads to the creation of an I-Thou relationship (Buber 2010) with her baby.

There is, however, another way in which women open themselves up in motherhood. An existential space (Deurzen 2009) is created as the mother becomes more open to her existence. This existential space is linked to the losses highlighted by Jacobsen (2006). In a crisis something is inevitably lost from an individual's old way of living. For mothers this is particularly evident as their lives have become unfamiliar and in some cases unrecognisable, with changes to their normal routines, their relationships to others and to themselves and more importantly, changes to their whole worldview. These losses, however, keenly they are felt, allow for an opening up of the existential space. This was illustrated by Eleanor, a research participant, who stated, 'so you just get stripped back to nothing, where you count for nothing and the only important thing is looking after this baby' (Arnold-Baker 2015: 149). In order for something new to be born there needs to be a letting go of the old; the existential space allows for the creation of something new. Mothers, unshackled from their previous lives and selves, can re-create a sense of themselves as they expand into the space that is afforded by their freedom (Deurzen 2009). Kristeva (2002) describes motherhood as the true creative act and whilst the ability to create another human being is truly miraculous, the woman is also creating herself as a mother. Mother and baby are created together, they are intrinsically linked, one cannot exist without the other. There is something unique about this experience of motherhood which challenges a woman in this way.

Developing an Existential Understanding of Motherhood

The chapters presented in this book bring together the most recent and up to date qualitative, existential research into motherhood and the maternal experience. All the research was conducted at NSPC, London, as part of joint doctoral programmes in counselling psychology and psychotherapy with Middlesex University. The research is distinctive in its existential analysis which offers a unique lens through which motherhood can be examined and understood.

However, the book is also limited by the focus taken in this research in that it does not cover a more diverse range of maternal experience, such as adoptive, teenage, single, lesbian, Trans, or neuroatypical mothers. Sadly, a fuller exploration of the diversity of the motherhood experience is outside the scope of this book and would benefit a book of its own. The research on which this book is based has also mainly focused on the experience of early motherhood and is therefore limited in that it does not address how the maternal experience changes over time nor does it explore the struggles mothers often feel when their children leave home. It would be impossible to do justice to the diversity and complexity of the motherhood experience in one book, or even to capture the multiple ways in which women can be mothers. This book therefore offers an investigation of a cis-gendered experience of motherhood, and whilst this may be regarded as offering a normative view of motherhood, the existential perspective that is utilised aims to elucidate that despite the diversity of experience, there are fundamental aspects of human existence that all mothers share. These existential aspects of human existence transcend the diverse range of ontic experience and offer an understanding of how motherhood highlights elements of our human condition. This philosophical approach also aims to challenge the normative discourse and offer women a new way of thinking about their motherhood experience.

The book is divided into four sections, where each section provides a different viewpoint from which to understand the maternal experience and the existential crisis that it evokes. The first section explores the philosophical tensions that are inherent in motherhood. This section highlights how maternity brings forth a new awareness of life, either in terms of our existence, our embodiment, our sense of responsibility or freedom or our sense of not understanding our current experience.

The second section explores maternal mental health and the personal crisis some mothers experience. Price (1988) elucidated in her work the emotional challenges that confront women when they become mothers, these challenges can often overwhelm mothers in such a way that their mental health suffers. This section examines the trauma that mothers of premature babies' experience in their first year after hospital discharge. It also provides a new understanding of postnatal depression both for the mother but also from the fathers' perspective of supporting a partner who is experiencing PND.

The third section focuses on the social crisis of motherhood and how society impacts on the mothers' experience and creates a social crisis for women. This section examines the social contexts into which mothers find themselves *thrown*. This includes a chapter on the experience of second-generation Ghanaian migrant mothers, which offers a cross-cultural perspective on how culture impacts the mothering journey and the mothers' identity. The mothers' experience of the traumatic loss of their child is also explored in this section. With the final two chapters grappling with the societal impact of 'choosing' motherhood, either because the woman is confronted with this maternal choice on reaching the age of 30 and discovering her freedom is constrained by her 'biological clock' or a woman chooses to remain child-free. Both chapters explore this nature of choice from opposing positions to highlight the tensions women face, whilst also elucidating the social tensions that arise from the concept of 'mother'.

The final section demonstrates how existential therapy can be utilised in working with the existential crisis of motherhood. An art-based approach to working with mothers' emotions, grounded in phenomenological research is offered as a way of helping mothers access and express emotions arising from their postnatal experience. A framework for existential therapeutic group work is also proposed as a way of guiding and helping women explore the four dimensions of their motherhood experience. The importance of being able to share experiences openly and honestly with like-minded mothers has been shown to be crucial in helping mothers reset themselves emotionally as a way of coping with the challenge's motherhood brings (Arnold-Baker 2015). The book concludes by drawing together the many threads and existential themes running throughout the different chapters. It explores the concept of existential courage that is needed to overcome the challenges posed by the existential crisis of motherhood. The final chapter also proposes a set of guiding principles to consider when working therapeutically with mothers, or indeed for mothers to contemplate for themselves as a way of reflecting on their motherhood journeys.

Most of the chapters are based on phenomenological research, using either Interpretative Phenomenological Analysis (IPA) (Smith et al. 2009), van Manen's (1990) lived experience method or Structural Existential Analysis (SEA) (Deurzen 2014). The remaining chapters are based on the extensive experience of the authors who have worked with mothers for many years. The names, and any identifying details of the participants, have been changed to protect the anonymity of the mothers who freely consented to giving voice to their experience; for which we are all grateful. Without their contributions our knowledge and understanding of the existential crisis of motherhood would be that much poorer.

References

Arnold-Baker, C. (2015). *How Becoming a Mother involves a Confrontation with Existence: An Existential-Phenomenological Exploration of the Experience of Early Motherhood* (Doctoral thesis, Middlesex University/New School of Psychotherapy and Counselling). http://eprints.mdx.ac.uk/18278/.

Arnold-Baker, C. (2019). The Public-Private Paradox: An Existential Exploration of Mothers in Society. *Self & Society, 47*(1) (Spring), 7–13.
Arnold-Baker, C., & Donaghy, M. (2005). Procreation. In E. van Deurzen & C. Arnold-Baker (Eds.), *Existential Perspectives on Human Issues*. London: Palgrave Macmillan.
Bollnow, O. (1959). Existenzphilosophie und Pädagogik. In Jacobsen, B. (2006). The Life Crisis in a Existential Perspective: Can Trauma and Crisis be Seen as an Aid in Personal Development? *Existential Analysis: Journal of the Society for Existential Analysis, 17*(1), 39–54.
Buber, M. (2010 [1937]). *I and Thou* (R. G. Smith, Trans). London: Continuum.
Collins Concise English Dictionary. (1993). 3rd ed., Harper Collins Publishers: Aylesbury.
Frankl, V. E. (1964). *Man's Search for Meaning*. London: Hodder and Stoughton.
Garland, V. (2019). *'Being-in-the-World' as a Mother Hermeneutic-Phenomenological Exploration of Lived Experiences of Eight New Mothers' Transition to Motherhood Within the Theoretical Frame of 'Four Dimensions of Existence'*. Degree of Doctor of Counselling Psychology, Middlesex University Repository.
Heidegger, M. (1962 [1927]). *Being and Time* (J. Macquarrie & E. S. Robinson, Trans.). Malden, MA and Oxford: Blackwell.
Jacobsen, B. (2006). The Life Crisis in a Existential Perspective: Can Trauma and Crisis be Seen as an Aid in Personal Development? *Existential Analysis: Journal of the Society for Existential Analysis, 17*(1), 39–54.
Jaspers, K. (1951). *The Way to Wisdom* (R. Manheim, Trans.). New Haven, CT and London: Yale University Press.
Kierkegaard, S. (1844). *Concept of Dread* (W. Lowrie, Trans.). Princeton: Princeton University Press.
Kierkegaard, S. (1962). *Works of Love* (H. V. & E. H. Hong, Trans.). London: Collins.
Kristeva, J. (2002). Maternity, Feminism and Female Sexuality. In K. Oliver (Ed.), *The Portable Kristeva*. New York: Columbia University Press.
Kruckman, L. D. (1992). Rituals and Support: An Anthropological View of Postpartum Depression. In J. A. Hamilton & P. N. Harberger (Eds.), *Postpartum Psychiatric Illness: A Picture Puzzle*. Philadelphia: University of Pennsylvania.

McCarthy, J. (2015). *A Body-Changing Event? Exploring First-Time Mothers' Embodied Experiences in the Post-Natal Period: A Hermeneutic-Phenomenological Study* (Doctoral thesis). University of Middlesex Repository.

Monk, H. (2013). Marketing Mothering as 'Crisis': Professions Saving us from the 'Danger' of Becoming Mothers. *Journal of Prenatal and Perinatal Psychology and Health, 27*(3) (Spring), 180–192.

Price, J. (1988). *Motherhood: What it Does to Your Mind*. London: Pandora.

Prinds, C., Hvidt, N.C., Mogensen, O., & Buus, N. (2013). *Making Existential Meaning in Transition to Motherhood: A Scoping Review*. Midwifery. http://dx.doi.org/10.1016/j.midw.2013.06.021.

Raphael, D. (Ed.). (1975). *Being Female: Reproduction, Power, and Change*. The Hague: Mouton Publishers.

Sartre, J.-P. (1943). *Being and Nothingness*. London: Routledge.

Smith, J., Flowers, P., & Larkin, M. (2009). *Interpretative Phenomenological Analysis: Theory, Method and Research*. London: Sage.

Stadlen, N. (2005). *What Mothers Do: Especially When it Looks Like Nothing*. London: Piatkus.

Stadlen, N. (2011). *How Mothers Love and How Relationships are Born*. London: Piatkus.

Stern, D., Bruschweiler-Stern, N., & Freeland, A. (1998). *The Birth of a Mother*. London: Bloomsbury Publishing.

van Deurzen, E. (2009). *Psychotherapy and the Quest for Happiness*. London: Sage.

van Deurzen, E. (2014). Structural Existential Analysis (SEA): A Phenomenological Research Method for Counselling Psychology. *Counselling Psychology Review, 29*(2) (June), 70–83.

van Gennep, A. (2004). *The Rites of Passage* (M. B. Vizedom & G. L., Trans.). Caffee. London: Routledge.

van Manen, M. (1990). *Researching Lived Experience: Human Science for an Action Sensitive Pedagogy*. New York: State University of New York Press.

2

Confronting Existence: The Existential Dimensions of Becoming a Mother

Claire Arnold-Baker

Introduction

Motherhood stops you in your tracks—'It is like being hit by a train, but in a good way' (Arnold-Baker 2015: 135) said Georgina, describing her experience of becoming a mother. This graphic image conjured up by Georgina encapsulates much of the complexity of motherhood. The emotions and feelings that are induced are often paradoxical, but there is also a force and a strength to the experience. It is an experience so powerful that it not only stops a woman in her tracks, but one that leads to a process of re-evaluation of herself and her life, which takes place during the first year and beyond.

Life changes completely and forever once a woman becomes a mother. There are many shifts that the mother has to undergo in her way of living during this transition, to incorporate her new baby into her life. Some of

C. Arnold-Baker (✉)
The New School of Psychotherapy and Counselling, London, UK
e-mail: claire@nspc.org.uk

C. Arnold-Baker (ed.), *The Existential Crisis of Motherhood*,
https://doi.org/10.1007/978-3-030-56499-5_2

these shifts are of a more practical nature and are therefore more noticeable, for example, changes to the mother's body or to the way in which she organises her day and life so that she can attend to her baby's needs. What is less noticeable and what this chapter aims to elucidate, are some of the more philosophical or existential issues that mothers are faced with, such as her mortality, temporality, relationships, identity, responsibility, freedom, choice and the unknown. These involve ontological shifts in a mother's way of *Being* which in turn will affect the way in which she understands life in general and her own existence in particular.

Whilst there has been a wealth of research and literature, from a variety of theoretical approaches, which have focused on many different aspects of the transition to motherhood, such as maternal identity (Smith 1994), social support (Goldstein et al. 1996) and the emotional response to motherhood (Price 1988), very little research has been conducted on the transition to motherhood from an existential perspective. Prinds et al. (2013) are most notable in addressing this gap with their scoping review of previous motherhood research, in which they conclude that 'becoming a mother is a significant life event. It is a transition in life, where existential considerations regarding the meaning of life are reinvigorated' (Prinds et al. 2013: 2).

The existential dimensions of this life changing transition are therefore important to articulate if we are to gain a deeper understanding of the motherhood experience. These dimensions form the existential ground upon which mothers' experiences are built. An understanding of the ontological structures of motherhood will explicate the enormity of the experience that becoming a mother is for a woman. A four-dimensional perspective, as conceived by Binswanger (1946), later refined by Deurzen (2012) and utilised in Prinds et al.'s (2013) research, also enables a wholistic view of the mother's life to emerge. The four dimensions: the physical or *Umwelt*; the social or *Mitwelt*; the personal or *Eigenwelt*; and the spiritual or *Uberwelt* dimensions [a further description of which can be found in Chapter 15], each provides a different emphasis on an individual's experience. The distinct dimensions present different challenges or struggles; unique tensions that mothers are faced with. For the most part these challenges are not consciously articulated by the mother and are instead felt as a sense of unease, anxiety or worry. If these challenges become too great, then the mother may slip into a depression or despair. However, an acknowledgement of the existential elements of motherhood demonstrates its complexity as a multi-dimensional experience, with inherent tensions and struggles on different levels. The motherhood experience in all its diversity begins to make more sense when women realise the ways in which they are being confronted by the givens of existence.

The Physical Dimension or Umwelt

Motherhood begins as an embodied experience. The physical act of conception and the resulting development of the foetus mean that a women's first experience of being a mother is through her body. The domination of the embodied experience continues in early motherhood with birth, breastfeeding and the postnatal body. Yet by the end of the first year there is a move in focus away from the embodied experience towards a process of making sense of the maternal experience in its entirety. At the end of the first year of motherhood, my findings demonstrated that the physical dimension of a mothers' existence, centred on her experience of temporality and time. The sense of her past, present and future but also the mother's experience of lived time.

Time and Temporarily: Living in the Present

In the first year of motherhood, mothers live mainly in the present; living from moment to moment. Their lives become more immediate and their focus is on what is happening right now or what needs to happen next.

The mothers' temporal sphere has narrowed and restricted so that it is now centred on the present and the immediate past and immediate future. This narrowing of temporality is not just 'because there's a lot more to deal with in the present' as Abigail states (Arnold-Baker 2015: 123); but rather it emerges from an urgent need for mothers to keep their babies' needs at the forefront of their attention. The vulnerability of the baby brings an urgency that is needed for its' survival.

However, this temporal shift has another existential dimension to it, that of spatiality. The mother's spatiality begins to alter in pregnancy. Her body schema adapts both externally, as her body takes up more space in the world as the baby develops and grows, but also internally, as the mother creates psychological and emotional space to allow for her to care for her baby and accept him into her life. However, it can be argued that there is a third aspect of spatiality which opens up during this period, and that is existential space. Existential space is created when mothers open themselves up to the new possibilities of their, and their babies, existence and this allows for this narrowing of temporality. The newness of the mother's situation and the importance of her baby do not allow for a wider focus.

Minkowsky (1933) conceptualised the present as the 'zone of activity' and this describes early motherhood well. Mothers are very active in the care of their babies, with all the associated activities that this involves. The present is also the sphere of 'being-with' (Heidegger 1962), which situates mothers in relationship with their immediate world, in this case the world of their babies. This leads to mothers being both relational and active in their care of their babies.

The concept of time also changes for mothers. My findings showed that they moved from *experienced time* our 'objectified, thought time', i.e. how we might think about time, or how our day, week, month and year is divided up, to *lived time*, which is 'the real inner time-happening' (Binswanger 1958: 301). The mothers felt that time itself had sped up. Everything felt new and constantly changing as their babies were developing and growing so fast. This also led to a feeling of immediacy or urgency. The normal structures and routines of the mothers' days were also no longer possible, as they now followed the rhythm of their babies, which often felt random and without structure. Beth articulated it as;

> It was weird, that whole kind of day and night, having no concept, it could be three in the morning and you're doing stuff and you're awake as if it's two in the afternoon. But I accepted that was the way it was. The whole, it doesn't matter, your life is in three or four hour cycles and that's just sort of the way it is. (Arnold-Baker 2015: 123)

These changes to the mothers' experience of time and temporality contributed to the feeling that motherhood was all-consuming. There was no space or time for mothers to be concerned with anything else, even attending to their own basic needs. Their whole *Being* was directed towards taking care of their babies. This meant there was little opportunity for the mothers to process what they were experiencing or to make sense of their motherhood experience. Abigail encapsulated this when she said;

> Babies just take up all of your thoughts and all of your days so you don't get time to kind of dwell on other things. (ibid., 124)

In order to make sense of our experience, we need to be able to reflect on what Heidegger (1962) termed the three *ecstasies* of time which form the life cycle of existence: being-ahead-of-oneself (future), having-been (past) and being-with (present). Being caught up in the present, with no time or space to contemplate ourselves or our lives means that it is difficult to reflect on what has been (past), in order to learn from or make sense of that experience. But it also means that it is hard for mothers to project themselves into *being-ahead-of-oneself*, the realm of the future. Not being able to reflect on the past or project into the future has the effect of keeping the mother in the realm of the present. This coupled with the all-consuming nature of motherhood leads to a *never-ending* quality of the motherhood experience. Christy summed it up when she said, 'I coped alright, but I just thought "God this is rubbish" [laughter], just like "O my God" and it feels never ending and it felt absolutely interminable' (Arnold-Baker 2015: 126). This never-ending quality explains why mothers can often feel that things will never change, or get better, why they can't see an end to the particular stage that they are facing. It is also emotionally exhausting and tiring, to be constantly living in the present in an all-consuming way. As Christy described, 'you don't see the constancy of it and how hard it is ... because it is the constant thinking about "right what am I doing next?"' (ibid., 125).

Life and Death

Gaining a sense of temporality in real time inevitably brings issues of life and death to the fore as it highlights how limited in time we are as individuals. Birth can sometimes feel a matter of life and death, both to baby and the mother. This is further compounded by how fragile the baby seems and in turn how fragile the mother may seem now she is faced with the importance of needing to stay alive for her child. Simone de Beauvoir (1997) also saw how temporality and mortality combined when a baby is born. The birth of a new generation means the mother moves along 'the great cycle of the species' to a middle generation, inextricably moving towards her own death. The mother moves from a *forgetfulness of Being* to a *Being-towards-Death* (Heidegger 1962), as she comes face to face with her own mortality. The realities of life and her existence are exposed in this mode of being and it reveals the mother's existential responsibility both to herself and to her baby.

The Social Dimension or Mitwelt

Life with a new baby thrusts the mother into a new social world: a world where relationships with other mothers and babies are newly formed, and where changes can occur with more established relationships. Namely the relationships with the mother's partner and her own mother but it may also extend to other family members, friends and work colleagues too. More importantly, however, is the developing relationship she creates with her baby. This unique relationship is one in which the mothers are heavily invested. It can at times feel one sided but nevertheless mothers direct themselves towards trying to understand their babies. In the process of understanding and responding to their babies needs they open themselves up to relating to their babies in new ways and this in turn effects the way they begin to see and understand their relationships with others.

Developing a Relationship with Her Baby

Perhaps the most difficult aspect for new mothers is how they try to make sense of and understand their babies' needs. Initially, this takes place at a non-verbal or embodied level, where mothers often feel that no real communication is taking place until the babies begin to respond through smiling or gurgling. In fact, mothers reported that mothering became easier for them once they could see responses from their babies. Although the interactions with a baby can feel one sided at first, a subtle form of communication is occurring between the mother and baby. This arises from the intentionality of the mother which is directed towards gaining an understanding of her baby through observing, responding and adapting to her baby. As Abigail explained;

> Early ideas about the kind of mother you'll be are reversed as you are learning about him… People say that you know your child best, but you haven't known them for that long and their communication is limited so you are just finding out, but sometimes you don't feel you know them at all… Yet how you deal with them is a lot more subconscious, you actually do know them quite well… what they prefer, you learn it together… But you don't consciously acknowledge to yourself what you have learnt. Only looking back do you realise how much you have learnt and how you've dealt with things together. (Arnold-Baker 2015: 116)

Abigail's description sums up the development of the relationship perfectly. It highlights the interactive nature of the mother-baby relationship (Stadlen 2005; Miller 2005) and how it is co-created between them as the mothers and their babies learn from each other.

The mother-baby relationship is dynamic and ongoing, it is a constantly changing process as mothers adapt and learn to be alongside their babies. Through this process, a relational bond grows, and love develops and deepens over time. Some mothers felt that they didn't get that first rush of love that they had expected after the birth and yet by the end of the first year the intensity of their feelings towards their babies were evident. Out of this deep connection, learning, love and openness, confidence grows, and mothers begin to feel more certain in their motherhood choices.

Connecting in this way involves a new mode of relating which opens up when a woman becomes a mother, again echoing Stadlen's (2005) observations. The mother moves to a *being-towards* mode of relating to her baby. For Heidegger this *being-towards* mode of being demonstrates concern and is a positive mode of relating (Heidegger 1996: 114). Through *being-towards* the mother's capacity to connect with her baby with care and concern opens up. She takes care of her baby, but not in a way in which she sees her baby as simply an object that needs looking after, but rather she is trying to understand her baby at a much deeper level. This type of relating is similar to Buber's (2000) *I-Thou* relating where the mother gives herself fully over to meeting her baby. Seeking to understand her baby's whole being by being open, receptive and attentive. Previous authors have described this mode of being as 'expert listening' (Levin 1989) or creating '*heartroom*' (Stadlen 2011). However, there is a mutuality in the relationship as Buber believed that babies also have an 'inborn Thou', an instinct to establish a relation, which turns into mutual relation or 'tenderness' (Buber 2000: 39). This can be understood as primordial intersubjectivity (Crossley 1996), a connection which is created in the space between the mother and baby. This connection, which develops out of intentionality, is needed in order for both to understand each other but there is also a need for mutual recognition.

Understanding Others

In the process of trying to understand their babies, the mothers described how they became more understanding of others and how their relationships to their partners and their own mothers also changed in the process. The mothers reported seeing their childhood from a new perspective, causing them to begin to reflect on their mothers and what it might have been like for them. The mothers were also more understanding of their partners, acknowledging how important this relationship was and how much they needed their partner's support. But the mothers were also concerned about how their partners were experiencing becoming co-parents and were aware of the challenges new parenthood brought to them both.

It is evident that when mothers enter a *being-towards* mode of relating they are not only opening themselves up to allow their baby to become central to their lives but this opening up extends to their other social relationships too. They became more understanding of others as they begin connecting to them in new ways too. Laney et al. (2014) understood this as demonstrating how mothers' selves expanded relationally as they become more open to others.

The Personal Dimension or Eigenwelt

Motherhood is a defining moment in a woman's life. It heralds in a new way of being and living and is a new stage in her life's journey. As Prinds et al note, the Eigenwelt 'confronts us with life events that put our inner self at stake' (Prinds et al. 2013: 18). Mothers are confronted with conflicting experiences, paradoxical feelings and uncertainty about themselves and their role of being a mother. All these aspects must be negotiated and re-negotiated as mothers make sense of what has happened to them. What emerges is a new sense of themselves as a mother: their maternal identity.

Life Is Different

The main tenet of this theme was how different the new mother's life had become. The mothers felt they had entered a whole new world, which was so different from their pre-baby days that they felt they could not really prepare for it. The expectations they had before the birth did not match up with the reality of the lived experience of motherhood. As Georgina said 'you had pre-conceptions of what it's going to be like and it's nothing like that. It's nothing. Not in a bad way. But it's nothing, nothing, like you would expect' (Arnold-Baker 2015: 134).

The babies consumed all their time and their thoughts so that there was no space for the new mothers to reassess their expectations or get a sense of what motherhood meant to them. Whilst this allowed the mothers to remain open and develop their own style of mothering, it can also be a very daunting and anxiety provoking experience as there is no familiar territory for them to stand firmly upon. They have entered a new world which felt like their life was starting over again with the birth. So much so that their previous life felt like it was in the distant past and didn't exist anymore. Part of this was because their babies have become central to their lives and their world changes to accommodate this shift. This shift in focus and lived experience also reflects a shift in priorities so that their babies and the life they are creating for their family becomes paramount. The mothers' previous way of living, although integral to them, became less important at this time. Their previous life felt more distant as they were now taken up with this new and all-consuming stage. Dani explained, 'Now I look back and think I can't ever imagine what time was like without her being here' (ibid., 136). All this can be experienced as a shock to the mothers who can't quite believe how different their lives had become. As Eleanor says 'I think it's like you're just in shell-shock. I think it takes a while to process what happened' (ibid., 139).

Adopting a Motherhood Identity

Inevitably, the changes that occurred to the mothers' life after the birth of their babies, to their relationships and to their priorities brought about a shift in how they also saw themselves. This shift, however, did not happen automatically directly after the birth. Instead mothers experienced a time where they had conflicting feelings about themselves and their sense of being a mother. For the mothers in my study there were four aspects to the motherhood identity; *not feeling different, not feeling like a mother*, *motherhood identity* and *important role*.

Initially, the women had an expectation that they would feel different about themselves when they became mothers, but surprisingly, they still felt the same as they did before the birth. Yet at the same time, they acknowledged that their lives were completely different and so much had changed. Fiona tried to express these contradictory feelings, 'I still think I'm me. I can easily switch off the mum – well I don't ever switch off being a mum' (ibid., 151). The mothers were holding the tension between the old and the new. There was a feeling of relief and surprise to feel the same and to have that continued sense of themselves. But there was also surprise that they didn't feel different, because their lives had changed so dramatically.

This tension was also confounded by a sense that the women did not feel like mothers. Their image or expectation of being a mother did not correspond to their experience of motherhood. Abigail summed it up as 'I'm not feeling what I'm supposed to be feeling as mothers' (ibid., 146). Beth said she had 'connotations on what a mother is and I don't feel like that ...I just think mothers just seem more established, being in control and being authoritative with children' (ibid., 146). Georgina felt she had preconceptions of mothers being weak and Fiona thought that being a mum meant you were boring. For Christy it was about being 'motherly' which was overprotective and overemotional and for Eleanor mothers were a bit frumpy and had a 'mumsiness' quality. All the mothers experienced a gap between the image they had of what a mother was and their own experience of motherhood. Often these images were negative and were based on a media portrayal, social norms or their views about their own mothers (Arnold-Baker 2019a).

During the first year of motherhood, mothers were grappling with these conflicting feelings about themselves. Although each mother reported a different experience, they all described how their sense of themselves had changed. For some it was a case of adding a new aspect to their identity. For others it was a stripping back of their identity to nothing and then gradually building it back up again. They felt that they started from a position of nothingness and through their experience of caring for and looking after their babies got a sense of what being a mother meant to them. Their sense of themselves as mothers came from their experience and their interactions with their babies and with others.

Previous literature and research confirms this view that motherhood is a transition time in which the mother reorganises and transforms her self-identity (Stadlen 2005; Stern 1995); that selves are complex and changing constructs (Smith 1994; Miller 2005; Hollway 2010), which were actively developed and created out of mothers experience, their life histories and their relationships (Wetherell 2009). Mothers therefore undergo an ongoing process in their sense of identity which involves constant negotiation and renegotiation as the mothers interact and gain more experiences.

This understanding of the development of the maternal identity gives credence to an existential view of self (Arnold-Baker 2019b). Sartre (1943) was notable in saying that 'existence precedes essence', i.e. that we have to exist in the world first before we can make sense of who we are. From an existential perspective there is no notion of a fixed and solid concept of self, rather we are always in a process of becoming. Therefore, the self is more temporal and ever changing but it is also relational. Heidegger posits, that as *Being-in-the-world*, we are constantly in relation with others and these relations determine how we think about ourselves. Much of the maternal identity research has confirmed these temporal and relational aspects of identity transformation (Mead 1934; MacIntyre 1981; Carr 1986; Ricoeur 1992; Blumenthal 1999).

Becoming a mother, therefore, can be a confusing time for women. It is a time where they hold the tension between their old way of seeing their lives and themselves and their new experiences of being a mother. To begin with, they feel the same as they did and yet their lives have changed immeasurably. They don't feel like a 'mum' because the images they have of being a mother are different to how they feel. It takes time for all of this to come together and to be understood by mothers. They need to make sense of what being a mother means to them personally. As Butterfield (2010) stated, we are always more than the identity we possess and so a woman is always more than just a mother. Being a mother is just one aspect of each woman and their identities are continually changing and adapting to the world they are experiencing, creating and relating to.

The Spiritual Dimension or Uberwelt

The spiritual dimension represents the world of our values and beliefs, our ideal world and where we create meaning and make sense of our lives. Motherhood compels the new mother to face the unknown elements of life and her existential responsibility towards herself and her child. But the mothers' expectations were also challenged, leading to a reassessment of their priorities in life.

Responsibility

For some existential philosophers (Sartre 1943; De Beauvoir 1997) responsibility forms the backbone of our human condition. Sartre's premise is that to be human is to be wholly responsible for our lives and selves. As human beings we are fundamentally free to choose how we live, and to live we must make choices. Part of this freedom is that we are then responsible for those choices and for the life we lead. For the most part we are only responsible for ourselves and we make choices that primarily affect our lives, but which will of course have an impact on others around us.

Sartre and De Beauvoir, however, did not consider the responsibility towards another that comes with having a baby. Being totally responsible for the life of another, who is vulnerable, dependent and unable to make choices and effect change on their own, throws light on the very tenets of existence for mothers. Previously mothers may have been unaware of the extent to which their existence is determined by their choices and the responsibility they face for those choices. However, this is brought into sharp focus by the birth of their babies when they are suddenly confronted with the reality of existence and their part in it. The mothers in this study were very mindful of how their choices would impact themselves and their babies. The choices the mothers had to make at the beginning were urgent and important and often felt like a matter of life or death. The vulnerability of the baby also highlighted the vulnerability of life and the mother's own mortality.

The mothers in my study found the constant decision making difficult and very tiring. They were faced with the enormity of each decision. They were choosing for another and would be answerable for that choice. The mothers wanted to make the right decisions for their babies but were often unsure what the right decision was, or how those choices would affect the future. They faced the existential struggle, which is inherent in human existence, that we have to choose, but are blind to the consequences of those choices and it is only in retrospect that we can say whether a choice was a good one or not (Kierkegaard 1844). This is perhaps, the hardest aspect of motherhood; that awareness of having to make vital choices but without the experience or knowledge to back those choices up.

Worrying

This weight of responsibility leads to a feeling of anguish and worry for mothers. Mothers worry about anything new that they must undertake, how they will be able to cope or the safety of their baby. Mothers can often be dismissed for their worrying, that they worry *too much*. But as Stadlen states worry is actually motherly concern and being careful, as mothers haven't 'got enough experience to be able to assess risks accurately' (Stadlen 2005: 20). But worry also comes out of the fact that mothers start to see the world in its raw state. Where they become conscious of their freedom, their choices and their responsibility. Where they see the fragility of life and how uncertain and unknown the future can be. The worry that the mothers felt came from a place of concern and care that they had for their babies and from an awareness of the reality of existence.

Challenging Expectations and Facing the Unknown

Whilst freedom to choose is an essential aspect of our human existence, there are also limits to this freedom, our 'ultimate situations' (Jaspers 1951) and therefore our existence. Becoming a mother involves a confrontation with the unknown aspects of life. Many elements of the mother's previous life have changed as she is faced with this very different experience. For some mothers even their values, beliefs and expectations are called into question, meaning they have no firm foundations to fall back on. It can be unsettling for new mothers who want to do the best for their babies to be in a position of not knowing. Facing the unknown can also feel chaotic and mothers can often feel out of control. Some mothers try to impose some control onto their situation, whilst others realise that this is just not possible. This was the case for some of the mothers in my study. They recognised that as much as they wanted to feel in control, they were in a situation that was not controllable. Some mothers reported that they reached a place where they accepted that they were subject to chance and began to 'let go' of their previously held expectations and beliefs and began to learn to 'go with' their babies rather than against them. Christy summed it up by saying, 'so it's probably got to actually having [baby girl] and being out of control and it was that big shift in my expectations really, of how to deal with that' (Arnold-Baker 2015: 143).

These shifts in expectations mean a re-evaluation of life for the mothers, as they reassessed their beliefs in light of their new experiences. The mothers' values also changed as they began to value the family life they were creating. But this extended to outside the family too as the mothers realised how important their role was in passing on their values to their children and how they were creating new members of society. These changes in values and beliefs bring about a new purpose in life for the mothers as they gain a new understanding of what is important in their lives. What was once a priority, such as the mother's career and work, may now no longer hold true. For this moment, their babies have become their purpose in life, and it has given their life a new meaning.

The Ontological Structures of Motherhood

This chapter has sought to uncover the experiences and changes that occur in women when they become mothers. In each dimension of existence, the physical, social, personal and spiritual, mothers are confronted with essential aspects of human existence.

The new mother has much to grapple with. Pregnancy, birth and caring for a vulnerable newborn brings the mother's existence to the fore and she is confronted with life and death, both her own and her baby's. The new mother's temporality changes and narrows, as she is now living in the present and her experience of lived time becomes set to the baby's rhythm. The mother becomes actively *being-towards*, to enable her to form a relationship with her baby and this radiates out to her other relationships too. Becoming responsible for another, who is vulnerable and unable to choose for themselves highlights the mothers' personal freedom, her choices and the consequences of those choices. This responsibility can often feel enormous.

At the same time, the mother questions her very being as she tries to make sense of her new experiences and role. Both will have an impact on her sense of herself and her identity. These different elements will inevitably lead the mother to re-evaluate her values and beliefs which in turn will transform the mother's meaning and purpose in life.

An existential analysis of motherhood has revealed its ontological structures to be; temporality, *being-towards*, freedom and responsibility, identity, thrownness, mortality, meaning and purpose. These are represented in Fig. 2.1, where each dimension displays the existential challenge facing the mother. These existential aspects of motherhood are just as important for mothers to consider, as the physical and emotional transformations which take place. Motherhood, therefore, is not limited in its scope to bringing a new life into the world and caring for it, it involves so much more. The *thrownness* (Heidegger, 1962) that mothers experience means they are confronted by existence in its raw state. The

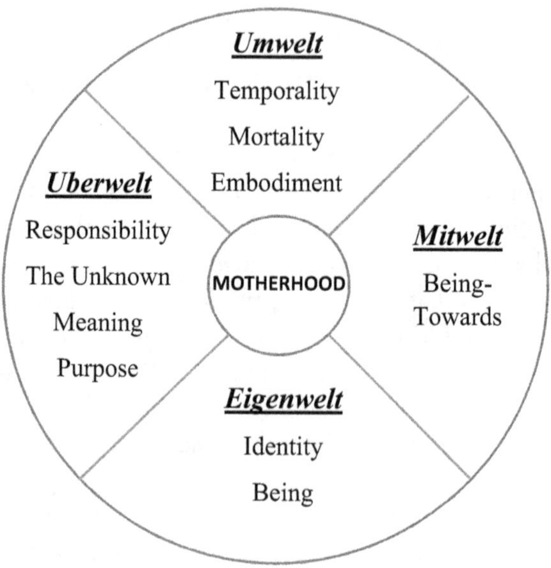

Fig. 2.1 The ontological structures of motherhood

reality of life becomes disclosed to them (Heidegger, 1962). In those early months, the new mother gains an awareness of existence as a whole and her place in it. She also has to confront the very notion of her own *Being* and how she makes sense of this in a changing, unfamiliar world. The transition to motherhood therefore is a transition in life, a window of awareness opens up for the mother and she sees existence in its raw state, this awareness will not always be so acute as it is in those early months of motherhood, but it is momentous enough for the mother to make significant changes in how she thinks about herself, her life and its meaning and purpose.

References

Arnold-Baker, C. (2015). *How Becoming a Mother involves a Confrontation with Existence: An Existential-Phenomenological Exploration of the Experience of Early Motherhood* (Doctoral thesis, Middlesex University/New School of Psychotherapy and Counselling). http://eprints.mdx.ac.uk/18278/.

Arnold-Baker, C. (2019a). The Public-Private Paradox: An Existential Exploration of Mothers in Society. *Self & Society, 47*(1) (Spring), 7–13.

Arnold-Baker, C. (2019b, July). The Process of Becoming: Maternal Identity in the Transition to Motherhood. *Existential Analysis, 30*(2), 260–274.

Binswanger, L. (1946). The Existential School of Thought. In R. May, et al. (Eds.), *Existence*. New York: Basic Books.

Binswanger, L. (1958). The Case of Ellen West. In R. May, E. Angel, & H. F. Ellenberger (Eds.), *Existence: A New Dimension in Psychiatry and Psychology*. New York: Basic Books.

Blumenthal, D. (1999). Representing the Divided Self. *Qualitative Inquiry, 5*(3), 377–392.

Buber, M. (2000). *I and Thou* (R. G. Smith, Trans.). New York: Scribner Classics.

Butterfield, E. (2010). 'Days and Nights of a New Mother': Existentialism in the Nursery. In S. Lintott (Ed.), *Motherhood: Philosophy for Everyone*. West Sussex: Wiley-Blackwell.

Carr, D. (1986). *Time, Narrative and History*. Bloomington: University of Indiana Press.

Crossley, N. (1996). *Intersubjectivity: The Fabric of Social Becoming*. London: Sage.

De Beauvoir, S. (1997). *The Second Sex*. London: Vintage.

Goldstein, L. H., Diener, M. L., & Mangelsdorf, S. C. (1996). Maternal Characteristics and Social Support Across the Transition to Motherhood: Associations with Maternal Behaviour. *Journal of Family Psychology, 10*(1), 60–71.

Heidegger, M. (1962). *Being and Time* (J. Macquarrie & E. S. Robinson, Trans.). New York: Harper & Row.

Heidegger, M. (1996). *Being and Time* (J. Stambaugh, Trans.). New York: SUNY Press.

Hollway, W. (2010). Relationality: The Intersubjective Foundations of Identity. In M. Wetherell & C. Talpade Mohanty (Eds.), *The Sage Handbook of Identities.* London: Sage.

Jaspers, K. (1951). *The Way to Wisdom* (R. Manheim, Trans.). New Haven, CT and London: Yale University Press.

Kierkegaard, S. (1980) *The Sickness unto Death* (H. V. & E. H. Hong, Trans.). Princeton: Princeton University Press.

Kierkegaard, S. (1844 [1980]). *The Concept of Anxiety*' (R. Thomte, Trans.). Princeton, NJ: Princeton University Press.

Laney, E. K., Carruthers, L., Hall, M. E. L., & Anderson, T. (2014). Expanding the Self: Motherhood and Identity Development in Faculty Women. *Journal of Family Issues, 35*(9), 1227–1251.

Levin, D. M. (1989). *The Listening Self*. London and New York: Routledge.

MacIntyre, A. (1981). *After Virtue*. Notre Dame: University of Notre Dame Press.

Mead, G. H. (1934). *Mind, Self and Society*. Chicago: University of Chicago.

Miller, T. (2005). *Making Sense of Motherhood: A Narrative Approach.* Cambridge: Cambridge University Press.

Minkowsky, E. (1933 [1994]). Findings in a Case of Schizophrenic Depression. In R. May et al. (Eds.), *Existence.* New York: Basic Books.

Price, J. (1988). *Motherhood: What It Does to Your Mind*. London: Pandora.

Prinds, C., Hvidt, N. C., Mogensen, O., & Buus, N. (2013). Making Existential Meaning in Transition to Motherhood: A Scoping Review. *Midwifery.* https://doi.org/10.1016/j.midw.2013.06.021.

Ricoeur, P. (1992). *Oneself as Another*. Chicago: University of Chicago Press.

Sartre, J.-P. (1943). *Being and Nothingness*. London: Routledge.

Smith, J. A. (1994, August). Reconstructing Selves: An Analysis of Discrepancies Between Women's Contemporaneous and Retrospective Accounts of the Transition to Motherhood. *British Journal of Psychology, 85*(3), 371–392.

Stadlen, N. (2005). *What Mothers Do: Especially When it Looks Like Nothing*. London: Piatkus.

Stadlen, N. (2011). *How Mothers Love and How Relationships are Born*. London: Piatkus.

Stern, D. (1995). *The Motherhood Constellation: A Unified View of Parent-Infant Psychotherapy*. London: Karnac Books.

van Deurzen, E. (2012). *Existential Counselling and Psychotherapy in Practice*. London: Sage.

Wetherell, M. (Ed.). (2009). *Theorizing Identities and Social Action*. London: Palgrave Macmillan.

3

The Corporeal Dimensions of Motherhood

Julie McCarthy

Introduction

This chapter is situated within Part 1 of this book since any consideration of corporeality necessarily enters the realms of philosophy. Philosophical discussions of embodiment have, until recently, failed to capture the fleshy nature of the lived body, offering more abstract understandings that speak *about* the body rather than *from* the body. The more discursive aspects of embodied experience have been well documented, with little attention paid to materiality, the body having been 'emptied of its organs' (Shildrick and Price 1999). Female embodied experience is only beginning to gain currency as a valid philosophical topic of investigation which is odd, given the singularly significant corporeal event that is pregnancy and birth.

In this chapter, I suggest that what constitutes knowledge about the maternal body needs to be renegotiated to include 'interior awareness' or 'kinaesthetic consciousness' (Rea 1977) and 'tacit knowing' (Polyani

J. McCarthy (✉)
The New School of Psychotherapy and Counselling, London, England, UK

C. Arnold-Baker (ed.), *The Existential Crisis of Motherhood*,
https://doi.org/10.1007/978-3-030-56499-5_3

1969), since if we curtail the tacit, we necessarily limit the possibilities of knowing. I also suggest that, in paying attention to our bodies it is possible to illuminate our understanding, not only of how we are in the world, but of *who* we are. This chapter therefore aims specifically to explore the centrality of maternal embodied experience to a new mother's sense of self. It explores whether embodied change in the post-natal period is indicative of larger elements of identity and investigates whether the body-self is irrevocably changed by motherhood.

Loss of Corporeal Autonomy

Changes to the pregnant body do not stop at birth. In many ways, the idea of a 'fourth trimester' does justice to the continuation of the body's adaptation to pregnancy and the woman's adaptation to her changing experience of embodiment. The post-birth body can be seen as an 'in-between' body, a liminal body subject to more nuanced readings of body image and corporeal ambiguity. There is a renegotiation of body boundaries that requires attention and adjustment: engorged breasts, cracked nipples, contracting uterus, stitched perineum, backache, headache following epidural anaesthesia, sleep deprivation—all require bodily adjustments (Neiterman 2012). These adjustments are part of the invisible work new mothers do whilst coping with the physical demands of caring for a newborn (feeding on demand, cradling for long periods, disrupted sleep).

> *Amanda*: All the shifts you have to make, they require a lot of work and some of it's hidden and some of it is very obvious so fundamentally every aspect—there isn't really an aspect of your life that's the same.

The physical aftermath of birth and the physical and emotional demands of early motherhood are a potentially overwhelming experience that can threaten any sense of autonomy over a body which has now taken second place to that of the baby. For a new mother, attending to her body's needs is a secondary consideration, a luxury. Tending to the unruly, messy, leaky, flabby post-natal body takes time and planning, commitment and dedication. Biologically there is a lot going on, internal organs are gradually settling back into place and shrinking to their original size;

hormones are in flux. Precisely at a time when a woman may need to attend to her body the most, she is physically and practically limited in her capacity to do so. The post-natal world is a world that has been tilted on its axis and post-natal embodied subjectivity is virgin territory: A new mother may therefore experience her body as no longer her own and her being-in-the-world as no longer autonomous.

> *Celeste*: For example, for the past twelve months since I had the baby it's been a case of everything goes on a priority list and the strictness and control, I had to let up on it.

Inherent in this loss of autonomy is the objectification of the mother's body which calls into question her sense of herself as usurped, squeezed out, discounted. Intrinsic to this is an underlying dissatisfaction with body shape and size which, during pregnancy, had been mediated and made more acceptable by the belief that bodily order and control will return as soon as the body has completed the project of pregnancy. The disorientating and sometimes overwhelming effects of a newborn on day-to-day life can shatter any self-made promises to take charge of diet and fitness regimes, even for the most self-disciplined and motivated of women.

> *Jen*: … actually the kind of priority is just existing and coping—the way I used to stay in shape was I'd do more physical activity, and obviously now there's not the time or opportunity.
>
> *Celeste*: You're so sleep deprived and it's such a big impact on your life that everything has a pecking order and the diet was low priority—you don't really have time to think, right, how many calories have I done?

Media coverage of celebrity mums 'racing back' (Roth et al. 2012) to slender, well-toned bodies with 'trim waists' and 'taut tummies' *in record time* propounds the ideological process of weight loss post-birth as a race—something to be achieved and celebrated. Achieving this represents a certain social status, the female body becoming a kind of 'currency' used for acceptance and integration into society (ibid.). In this way, the postpartum body is controlled through public ideologies of an 'ideal' body type and the postpartum body is deemed unacceptable and in need of a make-over. Whereas in pregnancy clothes are designed to 'show off' the pregnant form, after birth they are designed to 'cover you up' as if by way of an apology (Upton and Han 2003). The post-natal belly is not fit for public consumption since in Western culture 'fat' symbolises an impoverished 'self' lacking in sexuality, control and even morality. 'Fat' bodies-selves are not publicly visible or viable. To be 'fat' therefore is to fail at being a contemporary woman (Nash 2010, 2012) which perhaps explains why some mothers cling to a prior body or body image in an attempt at preserving a prior social status and sense of self.

> *Carol*: They're telling you that you shouldn't have a mark on you. They're telling you that you should spring back and they say that they think a mum is being selfish if she doesn't do her exercises and get her body back.

However, a mother without a mother's body, whose requirement or commission was that? (Dworkin and Wach 2013). It seems we have become convinced that these overhanging tummies, stretch-marked skin and scarred flesh are ugly and unsightly, signs that a woman has lost all control over her body and 'let herself go'. However, when viewed as part of the whole woman, mothers' bodies appear congruous and bear witness to the importance of redefining the materiality of the post-natal body by throwing off the blanket of shame that has been wrapped around the body of a mother to reveal the lived reality of embodied motherhood. The experience of loss of corporeal autonomy in the post-natal period could in this way be reduced.

Loss of Corporeal Integrity

Encountering the body for the first time after childbirth can be a deeply unsettling experience. Bodily sensations may be unlike anything feelingly known before as a new mother enters unchartered carnal territory. The body draws attention to itself in this alienated state. It calls us into itself, no longer a backdrop to our preoccupation with life. The body can feel out of sync and as a result our relationship with the world is out of sync, bodily changes having instigated a changed physiognomy of the world (van Manen 2014). Ordinarily, when bodily engaged in the world, we cease to notice our bodies. We fail to take notice of it since, as the means of our subjectivity, it is 'passed by in silence' (Sartre, [1943] 1969). It is only when the body call us, through pain, malfunction, illness or discomfort, that the body becomes a different entity, an object (van Manen 2014). Bodies or body parts become estranged, cut-off, distant, alien, foreign. The body can be felt to possess malevolent intent, attacking us, limiting our ambition for ourselves, killing us even. The body becomes prohibitive, standing in the way of one's being-in-the-world, hindering one's project, impeding Dasein.

> *Celeste*: I felt resentful towards my body, almost like 'why are you doing this?' … There are times when you are so frustrated that you feel completely detached from it and my body is a completely different entity and you're like 'stop doing this!'

New mothers can experience themselves as 'abject', as an unstable, leaking essence (Longhurst 2001, 2005). Material remnants of her body have been left behind—blood, amniotic fluid, placenta, umbilical cord, sometimes muscle and tissue, all extracted and disposed of. A new mother is materially altered by birth, literally transformed. The experience of physical vulnerability whilst shuffling around the maternity ward in flight socks, perhaps unable to stand upright due to the pain of abdominal or perineal stitches, the sensation of wetness due to blood, colostrum, milk or urine saturating gowns and bedclothes suggest a post-natal body that is synonymous with injury. Sensations such as hanging, dragging, tingling, searing, burning, stretching, tearing, throbbing, aching, pulsating, penetrating, undulating, sharp, flopping, wobbling, bulging, oozing, leaking, dripping, creaking and pounding can usher in feelings of bodily disintegration, fragmentation, alienation, dissociation and pain which underpin a loss of corporeal integrity.

> *Jen*: That area down there just feels kind of—it's like a wound, you know what I mean? You're just affected. I mean, I think I was almost too scared to look down there for a long time, so in a way I just left it.

For some new mothers this can be the experience of being in a body that no longer resonates with the self, which exudes pain and discomfort to such an extent that it no longer belongs. Body and self can seem divorced from each other, body parts split off, exorcised from a more healthy core. This new, aching blancmange of a body can be experienced as alien territory and uncanny alteration—unknown fleshy subjectivity. It is impossible to ignore the body, suppress its demands or hide from it; it is not easily separable from a sense of self and the world continues to be navigated through altered senses, altered bellies, hips, thighs, perineums and breasts.

> *Carol*: It was separate from me; It was a thing that hung on me for a while.

For many new mothers, there is an overarching sense of shock at embodying this new emptied flesh which no longer resonates with a prior sense of self (Oakley 1980; Bailey 2001; Way 2012; McCarthy 2015). This can be unexpected, unforeseen and unplanned for since post-natal bodies are secret bodies, private bodies. There is a sense that 'no-one tells you' with undertones of disbelief and betrayal for the newborn mother who feels duped by other, trusted, mothers who a priori knew her fate but failed to warn her. The embodied dimensions of birth can therefore catapult new mothers out of their corporeal comfort zone unarmed, feeling resentful, angry and confused.

> *Jen*: It's very weird, 'cos you almost kind of feel, I know, I mean I can't really articulate it very well, but you almost feel *tricked*… I think it is just totally glossed over … no-one goes into how it actually *feels*.
>
> *Carol*: It doesn't matter how many people tell you, until you've done it there's a difference. I wish I could go back and just warn myself.

There can be for some new mothers a fear that this liminal body represents the new normal, and that any connection to a prior, increasingly unfamiliar, functioning, socially acceptable body is lost.

Pain, discomfort, loss of function and changes to cosmetic appearance in the post-natal period are overlooked, downplayed or minimised as seemingly minor concerns against the more important work of motherhood. The expectation of going back to 'normal' is seen as a bonus rather than a given. Feelings of alienation from a prior body give rise to new mothers describing their bodies as functional rather than sentient, as a tool rather than a source of personal enjoyment (Bailey 2001).

Amanda: And it's being indulgent if you want to rectify something and no, it's not being indulgent. It's a level of functioning that I'd actually like to restore please!

In striving to meet social expectations of a return to normality (regardless of bodily state), mothers' bodily impressions and perceptions are dismissed, downplayed or muted in an attempt to keep up appearances (Bailey 2001; Way 2012; McCarthy 2015). This 'business-as-usual' front can be played out in the wake of even extreme physical pain and discomfort, the 'normal' body experienced as inaccessible in the face of every-day rituals of life such as cooking supper, doing the school run and keeping the house clean. These tasks merely give a semblance of normality lived through an embodied subjectivity that no longer feels integral to a sense of self. 'True' normality, however, is only restored through the subjective experience of getting the body 'back'.

Carol: I started to lose weight and everything started to go back to normal and I stopped looking at myself and thinking 'Oh, I hate myself!' and started looking at myself and going 'hello!'

Loss of Corporeal Identity

Birth being such a carnal event, it follows that in the post-natal period a woman is faced with exploring the relationship between her changing body and her identity as a new mother. This relationship is informed by public, private and professional discourses around pregnancy, birth and parenting. Society's preoccupation with an 'ideal' female body is transferred to expectations of what the early postpartum body *should* look like, suggesting the idea of an unchanging female body, interrupted briefly by pregnancy.

When a body no longer conforms to its previous (known) shape and no longer feels the same, moves in the same way or inhabits space in the same way, there is for a new mother the experience of her body as unrecognisable and distressing. There occurs a seismic shift in identity and with this a giddying sense of lost-ness and alienation. There is a disconnect from the body which undermines her ability to recognise herself. Only when her body starts to assume a more easily identifiable, socially sanctioned shape does she start to re-encounter herself again. In that moment of re-encounter there is a sense of belonging—of coming home to your body. A reconnection to a familiar self is made accessible through reconnection with a familiar body.

> *Carol*: I do feel I disappeared for a while … more and more now I look in the mirror and it's like I can see myself again. Before that, in the beginning [breaking down] I would look at myself and [unable to continue for a while] I was lost. I kept revising my body in a kind of, looking at the mirror and [sucking in her breath], yeah, can't deal with that yet.

A woman's body is therefore intrinsic to her sense of self. It is her display of femininity, of womanhood: how she moves, how her clothes hang on her, how toned her body looks are all implicated in whether or not she feels good about herself. A woman's body secures her a particular place in the world, secures her either admiration and applause or mockery and rejection. A changed body, especially when it overhangs, flops and sags, when it threatens the adoption of a 'fat' identity, invokes shame and self-loathing. A changed body robs a woman of her status, her self-belief.

> *Carol*: I didn't expect everything to be so saggy… I really did feel like a deflated balloon. The logic part of me is going I know this is going to take time to get back, but at the same time I'm like 'Oh my god! Someone's deflated me!'.

The loss of the old, familiar body can be emotionally overwhelming. What is lost is not only body confidence, but confidence in herself as a woman and as a mother. There transpires a mind/body split, a feeling of not being coherent, complete, at home—a physical distance from a body that was once still intrinsically known but now lost, a disconnect from the body-person that *was* and the body/person that *is*. Having to navigate the transition to motherhood in an altered body can be for some a deeply distressing experience. The body becomes a kind of subjective object, mine but not mine, functioning, but not as I know it, an unfamiliar vehicle in which to navigate a new material landscape.

> *Carol*: Sometimes I look at her and I think 'am I ruined? Is this what I'm going to be now?'

There ensues an alienated objectification of the body, a disembodied conceptualisation of the body as 'not me' that positions the body as 'other' and reinforces Cartesian notions of a dichotomy between subject and object, self and other, body and mind, flesh and consciousness. The body is conceptualised in this way as either a transparent mediator for our projects or an objectified and alienated resistance to being-in-the-world.

> *Amanda*: I do feel vulnerable with this breast ... well, this is not a feeding breast and now it's disgusting it's not a sexual breast [laughing] it has no function, it's just this appendage... it's a thing I have to see to or it's something I have to look after. But it's not really serving it's purpose, I've just got to stop it causing me grief, which is quite sad really.

The experience of bodily shame can exile new mothers from their taken-for-granted place in the world, rob them of their identity and change their social status. From an existential point of view, shame is predicated upon objectification, upon being seen or exposed, being caught in the 'look' of the Other (Sartre [1943] 1969). The look dis-embeds us from our world, distances us from our sense of self. In the look there is an awareness of the body as it is for the Other.

> *Carol*: I hated myself for it, really strangely. I would sit here and like [looking down at her breasts] *almost as if they were the enemy!*

Bodily shame can also be understood through the lens of 'the abject' (Kristeva 1982). To embody a maternal identity is to embody the abject, to embody filth and decay—especially so in the post-natal period, when internal fluids have been expelled: blood, mucus, placenta, milk—all of which transgress the borders of the symbolic and shake the very foundations of a stable and unified identity. Maternity therefore both inaugurates and demands the shaking up of taken-for-granted, assumed concrete, notions of selfhood which are always teetering on the brink of the abyss. Feelings of bodily disgust and rejection, as well as the requirements on a new mother to return to a former, whole, socially sanctioned body, is perhaps then fuelled by semiotic drives (sexuality, corporeality) which represent a danger to the stability of the subject being signified as abject. The abject attests to the psycho-social horror at the objects that transgress borders and boundaries—bodily fluids, wastes, refuse—and signify the subject's mortality. The body subject recoils from its own materiality. Interior matter, that which is alive, is deemed clean, but all that is expelled is imbued with filth and defilement (Grosz 1989). To embody the abject is therefore to embody the ever present threat to identity.

> *Carol*: Occasionally I would leak, and then it would be like, I can make enough to be embarrassing, but I can't make enough to feed my baby.

In rejecting the post-natal embodied self, something else fundamental to a mother's identity can become tarnished, eroded or lost—her sexuality. Alienation from, and rejection of, the physical body can render a new mother struggling to exist as a being-for-others, to share her physical body with her partner. Until the old, familiar, acceptable body returns she is existentially on hold, unable to truly, authentically exist as a fully embodied (sexual) being-in-the-world. The sexual self can go missing and with it a desire for the other. Physical, bodily intimacy is denied, and all carnal activity halted. In fact, some mothers find it difficult to describe themselves in sexual terms after birth, with an identification with 'someone's mum' rather than as a woman (Bailey 2001).

> *Charlotte*: It caused a massive wedge between us because he still wants to be physical with me but I hate him looking at me… all these bloody rolls of fat. And I hate that I'm pushing him away, but I can't bear him touching me.
>
> *Carol*: The physical side of myself, I couldn't bear to look at it and things felt different, sex felt different …

Perhaps because mothers' bodies have been freely made available to the Other, 'gifted' through an act of 'corporeal generosity' (Diprose 2002), there is a worry that their identity as women, rather than as mothers, is being eroded. However, since the body is a priori given in the creation of identity, being primarily social beings, our bodily existence therefore has the potential to create new possibilities for being through our embodied interaction with others. An altered identity in the post-natal period is therefore unavoidable in the wake of pregnancy, birth and breastfeeding and maternity can be regarded, not as a loss of self, but as a potent process in the creation of a new self (ibid.). Presumably, this involves a letting go of old notions of what it means to be an autonomous self and an openness to forming novel identities made possible through the relationship with the newborn. In this way, new motherhood can create opportunities for women to claim back a more potent sense of embodied agency and offers a more dynamic interpretation of an identity in flux.

The ontological dimensions of bodily concerns—concerns with cosmetic appearance, shape, size, function and damage—go far beyond surface or vain indulgences and strike at the very heart of the woman herself. A dialogue is invited here between the expectations placed upon a new mother (and her body) and the lived reality of embodied motherhood which can smash all notions of selfhood including self-image, self-efficacy and self-worth. However, it is in inviting an awareness of a subjectively displaced body, with curiosity rather than with objectification, that a mother can have the potential to experience her body as fulness rather than lack (Gadow 1980), positioning consciousness within the body in such a way that it is always experienced as *me*.

The Embodied Dimensions of Breastfeeding

Any consideration of post-natal embodiment would be incomplete without an exploration of the breastfeeding experience which I argue requires more than mere biological adaptation. Rather it poses new mothers with an existential challenge that can make or break perceived notions of (good) mothering. It is well documented that breastfeeding as an embodied practice is highly emotionally charged and has been associated with grief, sorrow and guilt (Battersby 2000; Ryan and Grace 2001; Shakespeare et al. 2004). It represents a complex subjective-corporeal activity which is also deeply embedded in sociocultural practices and is subject to moral and ethical scrutiny (Shaw 2004).

The intensely embodied nature of breastfeeding is subjectively experienced as either pleasurable, intimate and the means of emotional connection with the newborn or as difficult, unpleasant, disruptive and even violent or mutilating (Schmied and Lupton 2001). These polarities are underpinned by how easily a new mother adjusts to notions of blurred boundaries between self and other, and how easily she accepts the inextricable link between the body/self and that of her infant. For some mothers the connectedness to their babies whilst breastfeeding feels intimate and harmonious, whilst for others it threatens notions of identity that value autonomy, independence and control.

> *Jen*: So it is that thing—he comes back from work and says 'oh I missed her' and it's like, I'm looking forward to being able to miss her because at the moment I don't have that opportunity.

Changes to breasted experience (changes in breast shape and size, changes in function or purpose and changes in appearance) can initiate changes to personal and social identity. All usher in feelings of confusion, grief, loss, emptiness and lack (Young 1980). Whereas in the West, medicalised notions of the breast are as detachable, replaceable and dispensable parts, for a woman they are intrinsic to her sense of self. Bodies can be conceived of as 'fields of information' (Kirby 1997), the 'nature and function of muscles being coterminous with the nature and function of psychology' (Bartlett 2000:184) and breasts are potentially therefore 'fields of knowledge' (Kirby 1997). Thought of in this way, breastfeeding can be conceived of as a form of bodily intelligence, with breasts being 'thoughtful, knowledgeable, responsive, literate' (Bartlett 2002: 381). This inherent bodily knowledge is a primordial, pre-reflective, preverbal, pre-conceptual longing for the other, both bodies responding with immediacy and intimacy in a way that is 'interembodied' (Ryan et al. 2011). Breastfeeding mothers are therefore in a *matrescent state* Raphael (1973) which involves an intuitive kind of tacit knowing which is ontological in its origins. This primordial state is realised not only by thought and emotion, but by the body itself (Ryan et al. 2011).

Breastfeeding is both a physical and an emotional investment, an orientation towards motherhood, a statement of intent, a visible display of maternal power. Struggles with breastfeeding therefore undermine self-perceptions of bodily coherence which are tied up with notions of competence, autonomy, knowledge and control and which are synonymous with assumptions of 'good ' mothering. So intrinsic is the ability to breastfeed for those mothers who have invested in it, that any disruption can inaugurate a disrupted relationship between a mother and her body which can be deemed to have failed. A new mother can feel rage, anger, resentment and hatred towards the breast and there can be a sense of failure which is bound up with shame as 'faulty' body parts don't work, the maternal body having betrayed her as incompetent at motherhood. The dominant 'breast is best' discourse, so visible and powerful in its message, threatens to further damage a mother's perceived social position as a non-breastfeeding mother, undermining her sense of competency and self-confidence (McCarthy 2015).

Carol: You get lost in this haze, you know, and especially at the beginning, because I couldn't breastfeed, so you really get a sense of failure with that.

Amanda: … when you are feeding a minimum of eight times, that frequency of pain, that's what makes it so intense, so it's not like it will go in a few days, you're repeating something that is so painful but so important and so integral and so that's why it's such a toll on you emotionally … I just felt bombarded with it.

The physical sensations relating to breastfeeding—suctioning, leakage, latching on, let-down, engorgement and nipple pain—are usually confined to the private realm (Kelleher 2006). These can be experienced as a physical burden, a loss of agency, freedom, ego. For some mothers there can be a sense of suffocation within the breastfeeding relationship and an overwhelming sense of responsibility for the life of the baby. It can be difficult to achieve any physical distance from the baby, to shed parental responsibility for more than an hour or two or attain some sense of corporeal objectivity and separateness. The mother is 'on tap' and her bodily practices and routines have been disrupted, breasts having been distorted in sometimes undesirable ways. Breast sensations can be strange, heavy, painful or even excruciating as the breast is experienced as occupying a different space (Schmied and Lupton 2001). The breastfeeding mother and her baby are mutually co-dependent and it can be difficult to stand outside of the relationship to have a sense of difference, independence, selfhood. There is therefore a balancing act between the infant's and the woman's needs. This entails a movement from a bodily performance to an embodied relation with the infant and oneself, which might be understood as developing a new aspect of being for the new mother (Heidegger [1927] 1988).

Jen: … it's kind of the physical aspects of it—I am the one who gave birth to her and I am the one who's breastfeeding her, so there are those ties—I am the one who is ultimately responsible for her—there's that extra physical link.

Amanda: the most I've been away from him is five or six hours tops—but if you're bottle feeding you don't have that physical pull.

The breast is therefore an essential 'tool' of motherhood. It is also intrinsic to a woman's sexuality. The breast is functional, purposeful, intentional; it reaches out to the other extending pleasure, nourishment, comfort and arousal. It is a defining feature of womanhood—a source of both desire and fulfilment. The embodied experience of breastfeeding therefore evokes confusion. A taken-for-granted identity as 'lover', as sexual being, can be challenged by notions of the breast being used as a feeding tool. The physical experience of breastfeeding, how it feels to have a baby suck milk from the breast—the tingling, fizzing, electric, rhythmic pull on the nipple, the sensation or either pleasure, discomfort or pain and any association with sex may feel confusing and wrong. The sensory experience of breastfeeding can feel instinctively uncanny for some mothers. Breasts are confusing in that they shatter the border between motherhood and sexuality (Stearns 1999) so represent a 'scandal for patriarchy' (Young 1980). A mother is dichotomously conceptualised as either temptress or mother, Eve or the Virgin Mary, she cannot be both (Grosz 1989). Eve was led by her 'wayward desires', punished with mortality; The Virgin mother, by comparison, is compliant. She shows humility, self-abnegation and modesty. She is protective and nurturing. She is also sexless (ibid.). The Madonna must be a virgin and patriarchal logic separates motherhood from sexuality. This dichotomy of motherhood maps onto the dichotomy of good/bad, pure/impure (Young 1980). Only when love or attachment is 'defleshed' does it become good. Eroticism must be sublimated so that love can be perfected, fleshy eroticism being imbued with impurity and badness, the sexual body despised.

This can have a deeply unsettling effect on a mother's sense of self. With breastfeeding comes a more complicated breasted identity, women's breasts thought of as 'for' another, rather than for herself. Mothers can therefore feel usurped by the breastfeeding relationship and the conflicting and overwhelming demands on their ambiguous breasts. A mother's identity can be undermined by lactation and nurturance as she becomes a breast for the baby, a part-object, nothing more than a blank screen upon which are projected the needs of the infant (Kristeva 1982).

> *Charlotte*: I didn't like it. It just freaked me out a bit. I just remember thinking 'your boobs are for the husband'… and all of a sudden I had this baby drinking milk out of them and I was like, 'no way! I can't be dealing with that!'
>
> *Amanda*: I think for 'the boob' it's all those feelings you might have of your body not being your own or things happening beyond your control or serving other functions than what you are used to, sort of intensified.

Although feelings about breastfeeding are characterised by maternal ambivalence, the darker side of this material act can lead to negative consequences on the mother's ability to cope—cope with the pain, with the sedentary nature of it, with feeling exiled from public life, with being physically tied to a newborn and with not being in control of body shape and size (McCarthy 2015). The physical challenges of getting a newborn to latch on can leave a new mother feeling helpless, vulnerable, powerless and desperate. As breasts are handed over to be managed by another, there can be deep sensations of powerlessness and uselessness as breasts are handled, perhaps roughly, pulled, pushed, squeezed, nipped and squashed into babies' open mouths. Focusing on the mechanics of the act, the woman herself can get lost to the well-meaning midwife, health visitor or breastfeeding counsellor, a mere appendage to the all important breast which can shatter fragile mothering identities.

> *Amanda*: … and the midwife's attitude really stunk. She made me cry, twice. How she spoke to me was really not good and I remember her expressing colostrum and she really hurt me … and I remember yelping and it was not pleasant at all, it was very, very painful and so it went from excruciating to [no words to describe it].

Pain can also shatter illusions of the naturalness and convenience of breastfeeding as the lived, sensory reality of hot, searing, sharp, burning sensations can usher in fear and dread as the ordeal of feeding time approaches. This flies in the face of imagined visions of the infant at its mother's breast—serene, peaceful, content, dignified. What isn't fit for public viewing is the agony, horror and hell that can constitute the embodied reality of breastfeeding for some new mothers.

> *Amanda*: They don't tell you that when they go on about it—oh it's so convenient and it's so natural. And it is, it is all of those things, but … I was in a lot of pain to begin with, a lot of pain. I mean it makes me laugh now, my chest was literally covered from me digging my nails in. I mean, it's not the picture they have round the ward …

Conclusion

In this chapter, I tentatively suggested that the post-natal period for some new mothers can emerge as an embodied twilight zone characterised (albeit perhaps temporarily) by a sense of corporeal homelessness and ontological insecurity. The postpartum body is on its own biological and physiological journey and the way a woman makes sense of this journey can influence the mother she is in the process of becoming. Often women's bodies do go on to resemble their old, prior bodies, but this takes time, work and commitment on behalf of the mother. Often the body remains in a changed state—a 'mother's body' and this is either welcomed or rejected by the woman depending on her own particular embodied sense of self and identity in the world. For most, the body keeps the score, tells the story of a life created, formed, birthed and nurtured, indelibly and irrevocably carved into the flesh like graffiti—bellies, hips, breasts—and selves—all transformed.

References

Bailey, L. (2001). Gender Shows: First-Time Mothers and Embodied Selves. *Gender and Society, 15*, 110–127. https://doi.org/10.1177/089124301015001006.

Bartlett, A. (2000). Thinking Through Breasts: Writing Maternity. *Feminist Theory, 1*(2), 173–188.

Bartlett, A. (2002). Breastfeeding as Headwork: Corporeal Feminism and Meanings for Breastfeeding. *Women's Studies International Forum, 25*(3), 373–382.

Battersby, S. (2000). Breastfeeding and Bullying: Who's Putting the Pressure on? *Practicing Midwifery, 3,* 56–58.

Diprose, R. (2002). *Corporeal Generosity: On Giving with Nietzsche, Merleau—Ponty and Levinas.* Albany, NY: SUNY Press.

Dworkin, S. L., & Wachs, F. L. (2013). Getting Your Body Back: Postindustrial Fit Motherhood in Shape Fit Pregnancy Magazine. *Gender and Society, 18,* 160. https://doi.org/10.1177/0891243204266817.

Gadow, S. (1980). Body and Self: A Dialectic. *Journal of Medicine and Philosophy, 5*(3), 172–185.

Grosz, E. (1989). *Sexual Subversions: Three French Feminists.* Sydney, Welington, London and Boston: Allen and Unwin.

Heidegger, M. ([1927] 1988). *Being and Time* (MacQuarrie & E. Robinson, Trans. J.). Oxford: Blackwell.

Kelleher, C. M. (2006). The Physical Challenges of Early Breastfeeding. *Social Science and Medicine, 69,* 900–907. https://doi.org/10.1016/j.socscimed.2009.07.001.

Kirby, V. (1997). *Telling Flesh: The Substance of the Corporeal.* New York: Routledge.

Kristeva, J. (1982). *Powers of Horror: An Essay on Abjection.* New York: Colombia University Press.

Longhurst, R. (2001). Breaking Corporeal Boundaries: Pregnant Bodies in Public Places. In R. Holliday & J. Hassard (Eds.), *Contested Bodies.* London and New York: Routledge.

Longhurst, R. (2005). (Ad)dressing Pregnant Bodies in New Zealand: Clothing, Fashion, Subjectivities and Spatialities. *Gender, Place and Culture, 12*(4), 433–446. Available at http://dx.doi.org/10.1080/09663690500356842.

McCarthy, J. (2015). *A Body-Changing Event? Exploring First-Time Mothers' Embodied Experiences in the Post-Natal Period: A Hermeneutic-Phenomenological Study* (Doctoral thesis). University of Middlesex Repository.

Nash, M. (2010). Weighty Matters: Negotiating 'Fatness' And 'In-Betweenness' in Early Pregnancy. *Feminism & Psychology, 22,* 307–323. https://doi.org/10.1177/0959353512445361.

Nash, M. (2012). *Making 'Postmodern' Mothers: Pregnant Embodiment, Baby Bumps and Body Image.* Hampshire: Palgrave MacMillan.

Neiterman, E. (2012). 'Doing' Pregnancy: Pregnant Embodiment as Performance. *Women's Studies International Forum, 35*, 372–383. https://doi.org/10.1016/j.wsif.2012.07.004.

Oakley, A. (1980). *Women Confined: Towards a Sociology of Childbirth*. Oxford: Martin Robinson.

Polyani, M. (1969). *Knowing and Being*. Chicago: University of Chicago.

Raphael, D. (1973). *The Tender Gift: Breastfeeding*. New York: Schocken Books.

Rea, S. (1977). *Hatha Yoga as a Practice of Embodiment* (Unpublished MA Dissertation). University of California.

Roth, H., Homer, C., & Fenwick, J. (2012). "Bouncing back": How Australia's Leading Women's Magazines Portray the Postpartum 'Body'. *Women and Birth, 25*, 128–134. https://doi.org/10.1016/j.wombi.2011.08.004.

Ryan, K., Todres, L., & Alexander, J. (2011). Calling, Permission and Fulfilment: The Interembodied Experience of Breastfeeding. *Qualitative Health Research, 21*(6), 731–742.

Ryan, R. M., & Grace, V. M. (2001). Medicalisation and Women's Knowledge Construction of Understandings of Infant Feeding Decisions in Post WWII New Zealand. *Health Care for Women International, 22*(1), 483–500.

Sartre, J. P. ([1943] 1969). *Being and Nothingness* (E Barnes, Trans.). New York: Philosophy Library.

Schmied, V., & Lupton, D. (2001). Blurring the Boundaries: Breastfeeding and Maternal Subjectivity. *Sociology of Health & Illness, 23*(3), 234–250. https://doi.org/10.1111/1467-9566.00249.

Shakespeare, J., Blake, F., & Garcia, J. (2004). Breast-Feeding Difficulties Experienced by Women Taking Part in a Qualitative Study of Post-Natal Depression. *Midwifery, 20*, 251–260.

Shaw, R. (2004). Performing Breastfeeding: Embodiment, Ethics and the Maternal Subject. *Feminist Review, 78*, 99–116. https://doi.org/10.1057/palgrave.fr.9400186.

Shildrick, M., & Price, J. (Eds.). (1999). *Feminist Theory and the Body: A Reader*. New York: Routledge.

Stearns, C. A. (1999). Breastfeeding and the Good Maternal Body. *Gender & Society, 13*, 308–325. https://doi.org/10.1177/089124399013003003.

Upton, R. L., & Han, S. S. (2003). Maternity And its Discontents: 'Getting the Body Back' After Pregnancy. *Journal of Contemporary Ethnography, 32*, 670–692. https://doi.org/10.1177/0891241603257596.

Van Manen, M. (2014). *Phenomenology of Practice*. Walnut Creek, CA: Left Coast Press Inc.

Way, S. (2012). A Qualitative Study Exploring Women's Personal Experiences of Their Perineum After Childbirth: Expectations, Reality and Returning to Normality. *Midwifery, 28,* 712–719. https://doi.org/10.1016/j.midw.2011.08.011.

Young, I. M. (1980). *On Female Body Experience: Throwing Like a Girl and Other Essays*. New York: Churchill Livingstone.

4

Existential Responsibility of Motherhood

Victoria Garland

Motherhood

Defining the meaning of motherhood is a complex task. A Cambridge dictionary definition of a mother is 'a female parent', the definition of the English suffix-hood denoting 'state or condition of being, character or nature', and the definition of motherhood is 'the state of being a mother or the qualities or spirit of a mother'. Therefore, I can argue that when viewing the phenomenon of Motherhood through an existential lens, it can be described as a 'state or condition of being a mother' in other words, 'being-in-the-world' as a mother.

Arendell (2000) argued that mothering can be defined as an act of nurturing and caring for people, by women or men, whereas motherhood is one of the few universal roles assigned to women that has still remained a central aspect of most women's lives.

The above descriptions indicate that motherhood is much more than just a physical happening. There are many women who do not give birth

V. Garland (✉)
The New School of Psychotherapy and Counselling, London, UK

C. Arnold-Baker (ed.), *The Existential Crisis of Motherhood*,
https://doi.org/10.1007/978-3-030-56499-5_4

physically to a child yet have taken up the responsibility of being a mother in the most beautiful way. There are also women who become mothers by giving birth to children, but who do not accept responsibility for their children, and I could argue that, in so doing, they are not choosing motherhood. Further, O'Reilly (2010) argues that motherhood could take on different meanings for different mothers, birth mothers or adoptive mothers. Further, the meaning associated with motherhood varies across historical, sociocultural and political demographics. Allen (2006) addresses some historical and cross-cultural differences of motherhood. In his study, he demonstrates how different forces (feminist, historical or sociopolitical) could shape the meaning and practices of motherhood.

Transition to Motherhood

The phenomenon of motherhood is a subjective and complex concept to understand and interpret, and the transformative journey to motherhood can also be viewed and understood from many different perspectives, as it is a very individual experience for each woman.

Naomi Stadlen compares the transition to motherhood to emigrating to a new country, 'like emigrants, newly pregnant mothers have already left a familiar country and have started a journey towards somewhere new' (Stadlen 2004: 13). Further, she argues that this transformative journey begins when a woman makes the decision to have a child. As a woman is imagining, contemplating, and making plans for a life as a mother, she is already making a 'heartroom' for her imagined baby (ibid.: 18). Bergum also asked 'where does transformation begin? Is there a beginning?' (Bergum 1989: 39) suggesting that the decision to have a child is a transformative experience towards motherhood. With the birth of a child, or acceptance of a child into her life, a woman, now a mother, arrives to a new country called 'motherhood', where she has to understand and find her existential bearings, learn a new culture and language, learn how to be 'at home' in this new unfamiliar 'being-in-the-world' as a mother.

From a physiological perspective, giving birth to a child transforms a woman into a mother, but from an existential perspective, it is the acceptance of responsibility for that child that represents the foundational step into motherhood. An existential endeavour and an ontological transformation are at the heart of the transition into motherhood. This transition sees mothers face existential responsibility for themselves, as well as their child, across the four dimensions of existence, the physical, social, psychological and spiritual dimensions. As a result of choosing motherhood, a woman now a mother, is confronted with the awareness of her choices and how these form part of the process of re-constructing her Being on every dimension of existence, providing the potential for a more mindful, authentic way of 'Being-in-the-world-as-a-mother'.

The existential philosopher and writer Emmy van Deurzen (2005) tells us that the range and depth of human experience is so immense and diverse that it is impossible to do it justice, and she argues that the transition to motherhood is one of these unquantifiable experiences. Furthermore, as she suggests (Deurzen 1997), all our decisions and choices are influenced by a multitude of factors, including our past experiences, and expectations both present and future. The transitional road to motherhood is paved by determining factors such as history, culture and class, as well as hormonal, genetic and characteristic factors, and situational, contextual and interpersonal elements. Each individual possesses a unique combination or pattern of factors.

Therefore, the transition to motherhood is a phenomenon that needs to be examined and understood as a web of complex constellations. These have multiple bio-psycho-socio-spiritual influences which, in turn, position each woman as a unique being-in-the-world as a mother.

The transition to motherhood can be conceptualised as an existential voyage, from a life before motherhood where the woman is responsible for her own existence, to life as a mother where she must accept the responsibility for another (her child). Many researchers have highlighted the emotional, physical and psychological challenges of this journey, which entwine with the fundamental changes in the four dimensions of existence (Bergum 1989; McMahon 1995; Barclays et al. 1997; Barlow 1997; Stadlen 2004; Hartley 2005; Ruzza 2008; Woollett and Nicholson

1998; Darvil 2008; Vick and Haftin 2012; Prinds et al. 2013; Athan and Miller 2013; Arnold-Baker 2015).

Before motherhood, women experience themselves at the heart of their own life project, they have invested in their own education, career, social engagements, friendships, personal achievements, hobbies, interests, physical health, body image and so on. They make choices about what they want or need for themselves, and as a consequence take responsibility for their own 'me' project.

Responsibility in the Physical Dimension

The experience of childbirth ties women to the fundamental cycle of life: birth, death and re-birth. Through the experience of facing a new life, the woman, now a mother, is facing a death too. Life and death are connected biologically and psychologically, and by greeting one the new mother is greeting the other. Death is a primordial source of anxiety which new mothers experience when faced with the fragility of their children, the possibility of loss and the experience of responsibility for their children's survival (e.g. Price 1988; Bergum 1989; Stadlen 2004; Parker 2005; Hartley 2005; Prinds et al. 2013; Arnold-Baker 2015; Garland 2019). As Prinds et al. (2013) argue, it is through the experience of giving birth that a mother confronts the awareness of bodily limitations and possibilities, of her own and her infant's mortality and of a biological responsibility for sustaining life. Bergum (1989) also points out how through this awareness of responsibility for her child's life, a woman becomes conscious that something could go wrong: she is facing mortality, both her child's and her own. This heightened sense of mortal responsibility throws a mother into a renewed contemplation of how she should live (see also Arnold-Baker 2015). In light of the physical dimension of existence (Umwelt), this primal responsibility prompts a new mother's re-evaluation and reconstruction of her values, priorities and lifestyle of her *being-in-the-world* as a mother.

The transition to motherhood can therefore be thought of as an experience of being displaced, in an unanticipated way, from a sense of identification with the 'me' project, which creates an experience of loss:

loss of a familiar lifestyle, loss of choices for oneself, loss of individual responsibility and loss of autonomy and freedom (Barclays et al. 1997; Stadlen 2004; Darvil 2008; Hartley 2005; Prinds 2013; Arnold-Baker 2015; Garland 2019). The sheer weight of the responsibility for her child, as Stadlen (2004) describes, is overwhelming to the extent that a mother, no longer feels in charge of her own life since her child, by necessity, always comes first.

The role of motherhood delineates a defined line between a woman's past and her future (also see Arnold-Baker 2015). In the past, she was responsible only for her own existence; she lived within her 'me' project, when life was 'all about me' (Garland 2019). Now a woman accepts a new life project: her child, who becomes a central part of her being-in-the-world as a mother for the rest of her life.

In contrast to the ontic state before motherhood, a mother no longer lives and acts as if mortality is not a part of her existence. This new awareness (and attendant anxiety) of mortality, and attunement to the embodied limitations of being, shakes the mother out of an inauthentic way of being-in-the-world and prompts her towards a being that demands engagement with her existential givens (Bergum 1989; Leonard 1993; Smith-Pierce 1994; Hartley 2005). This more mindful awareness of death anxiety triggers a new level of experiencing responsibility for her child's life and her own, and provides a mother with the pathway to a more mindful mode of life, an authentic way of Being (Heidegger 1962).

Heidegger believed that there are two fundamental modes of existing in the world: a state of forgetfulness of being and a state of mindfulness of being. He states that when we immerse ourselves in the everyday diversions of life, we lose ourselves in the 'they' ('*das Man*') (Heidegger 1962). We live in a state of forgetfulness of being or in an inauthentic everyday mode of existence. Moreover, Heidegger argues that to move from a state of forgetfulness of Being into a mindfulness of Being we need to experience certain unalterable, irremediable conditions, or as Jaspers calls them, 'limit situations' (Jaspers 1994: 203). In normal situations, Jaspers asserts, one can make a comparison to other known situations and one can step in and out of them, whereas a limit situation is irrevocable; we cannot change it, we can only visualise it more clearly.

When stepping into the world of motherhood, women enter a limit situation, an irreversible, unfamiliar, unknown world. Thus, it could be argued that the journey to motherhood begins with defamiliarisation, in which women are dislodged from the place of 'at-homeness' (Heidegger 1962). Their relationship with the familiar world is profoundly shaken, and the everyday guidelines are suddenly stripped away; new mothers suddenly lose their sense of knowledge of the world, when the world that previously protected them from the anxiety of existential givens dissolves. Heidegger (1962) uses the term 'uncanny' (*Unheimlich*) to denote this experience of having lost contact with one's existential situation and the resulting feeling of not 'being-at-home-in-the-world'.

In other words, motherhood comprises a 'limit situation' (Jaspers 1994) or 'urgent experience' (Heidegger 1962), when the mother becomes existentially aware of her responsibility for the life and death of her children, and through this experience mothers enter a mindful or ontological mode of being (Heidegger1962).

According to Heidegger (1962) living in the mode of mindfulness of being or living in an authentic mode means to be continually aware of being, aware of its possibilities and limitations, aware of freedom, of choice and responsibility. Jacobsen (2007) stresses that to be responsible is to accept the consequences of your own actions. To be aware and to accept the responsibility for your choices is to be aware and accept the consequences of these choices. Choices therefore entail responsibility, awareness and acceptance. Sometimes, such a choice resembles a leap into the unknown.

According to Yalom (1980), the experience of defamiliarisation involves a variety of entities that provide structure and stability (e.g. rules, values and guidelines) and also time structures. In this new mode of being-in-the-world as mothers, women also experience a different awareness of time (clock time as opposed to existential time) and space. The experience of clock time changes from that of the familiar rules and guidelines: breakfast, lunch, dinner and night time, working time and free time, to the all consuming baby time.

To be able to take care of their babies' needs, mothers must be alert, aware of time, phenomenologically present in a here-and-now mode of time and space. Living in constant awareness of the presence of another being and continual alertness to your responsibility for that Being's survival and well-being stimulates the mother's perception that they are living with their children on their minds every moment of the day and night.

Stadlen (2004) speaks about how the responsibilities women hold before motherhood have the ability to be shared, passed on or even ignored. By comparison, the weight of a mother's responsibility is such that no-one can completely take her place. The mother is not just looking after her child, she is responsible for her child's well-being even in her absence.

Arnold-Baker (2015) reflects in her study how through learning to follow the rhythm of their baby's needs, a new mother adapts to a new sense of temporality. The mother's whole being is directed towards the care of her baby and through this peak awareness of life and death, the mother enters into a new relationship with existential time (Arnold-Baker 2015). They become aware of the temporality of existence, their own as well as their child's.

Living in this mode of continuous mindfulness of choices and responsibilities, and continual physical and psychological availability to the other (the child) is an exhausting experience. Most researchers have reflected on the mother's physical and emotional exhaustion, mostly during early motherhood (e.g. Barclays et al. 1997; Hartley 2005; Arnold-Baker 2015; Garland 2019). Stadlen points out that 'the tiredness of a new mother is in a league of its own' (Stadlen 2004: 110). Stadlen describes how mothers make choices over and over again to look after their children even at a cost to themselves in terms of fatigue, loss of sleep and declining personal interest in their own needs:

> Mothers might care for their babies at the cost of their own physical wellbeing. They themselves complain that they are not exercising choices…but of course they do have choices. They are exercising free will (Stadlen 2011: 98).

It could be argued that this mindfulness of choice and responsibility is one of the factors that leaves mothers so exhausted. However, this mindful mode of living, in spite of exhaustion and ambivalence, can also offer a mother the opportunity to live more authentically. For instance, the personal qualities that the mother becomes aware of in herself include the capacity for selflessness, perseverance and constant commitment in the face of overwhelming exhaustion.

Responsibility in the Social Dimension

When becoming a mother, a new relationship is formed with her child. She is defined by others and by herself in association with her child, as a mother. A woman is not only defined by who she is, a mother, but also how she is, her mothering, the way she is choosing to re-shape her way of being by connecting to her new environment or her new position in the world.

A number of studies have demonstrated that the transition to motherhood facilitates a gradual psychological opening to a profound social change, and encourages an active questioning of belonging; where values and priorities are re-evaluated, and relationships are transformed (e.g. Price 1988; Stadlen 2004; Adams et al. 2006; Sevon 2009; Butterfield 2010; Arnold-Baker 2015; Garland 2019).

Stadlen highlights that describing motherhood is describing 'being in a relationship' (Stadlen 2011: 14). As Lintott claims, 'this is not just any relationship – the mother and child are one being and two at the same time' (Lintotte 2011: 67). From Hartley's (2005) point of view, the relationship between a mother and a child is different to any other relationship in a woman's relational world. The child is central to the mother's existence, and as such they are not co-existent, they are not equal participants in a relationship because the baby totally relies on the mother, and the woman carries the baby, literally and ontologically, as part of her being-in-the-world. Hartley (2005) further argues that a mother's utter absorption in every mode of the child's being prompts her to turn her own being towards the child. This reconstructs her vision and relation to others (her partner, family, colleagues and friends). When a mother-child relationship enters the mother's social or relational world (*Mitwelt*), it squeezes into the dynamic of all her existing relationships, and as the result the shapes of these relationships are inevitably altered and re-evaluated. Therefore, her being-in-the-world as a mother and her being-with-others are re-constructed and her position within her life-world is recreated (Stadlen 2004; Sevon 2009).

Even though each woman experiences motherhood in her own unique way, Ehrenreich and English (1978) highlight that motherhood cannot be understood separately from the society in which it occurs. This complex experience manifests within core values and cultural principles that are inevitably internalised by members of any society. Butterfield (2010) highlights that the concept of the ideal mother (just as with the ideal feminine) is a social construct that varies historically and culturally. We are always fundamentally social; we live and move within the social realm via language and culture which give us the tools for understanding ourselves and the world we live in. The social realities of being a mother depend on those understandings; therefore, our freedom of choice is situational and the concept of being a mother is socially positioned in a specific way, within a social context in the world. However, each woman will choose how, and to what extent, she follows or swerves away from the 'normative, stereotypical expectations of motherhood' (Rich 1977:12), and decides for herself how will she mother.

Since a mothering role is culturally associated with responsibility, morality and caring, a woman who is seen as irresponsible towards her children would jeopardise far more than an inadequate role performance, it would be to portray herself as a bad mother. Butterfield describes the ambiguity of the human condition (Butterfield 2010: 74), in which we are never completely alone as individuals and we are also never completely lost in the social: the reality is in the tension of experiencing both at the same time. Therefore, to be a mother is to live within the boundaries that are determined by the society in which the mother is positioned, but a mother is still free to choose what being a mother will mean to her, how she will respond to the social script and how she will live this new identity as a mother within the larger social and cultural contexts (Butterfield 2010).

The new mother-child relationship instigates a 'being-toward' (Heidegger 1962) mode of relating and a more authentic position with regard to being-with-others. New mothers exercise their choice in the face of societal expectations, norms, demands and ethics. The weight of responsibility a mother feels for her child demands a reconstruction of her relationship with others (including her partner, her own mother, extended family and friendships) and herself.

Responsibility in the Personal Dimension

With the birth of a child, a motherhood identity is born. This identity is not chosen, it is given to a woman who gives birth to a child. However, choosing how to be a mother informs, shapes and develops that identity and this in turn generates changes to all the other identities in a woman's life. By choosing to take on the responsibility of motherhood, a woman is shaping her identity as a mother.

In reflecting on the new mothers' personal world (*Eigenwelt*), Vick and Hafting (2012) describe the loss of former identities in the transition to motherhood, and Barclays et al. (1997) similarly point to the loss of a sense of self. However, other researchers describe becoming a mother in terms of changes in the way women think about themselves (e.g. Arnold-Baker 2015), or in terms of the way in which the mother reorganises and transforms her self-identity (e.g. Stadlen 2004; Stern and Bruschweiler-Stern 1998; Prinds et al. 2013). Garland (2019) describes the transformation from a 'self-centered' relationship with oneself to a 'self-giving' one, in which the other (the child) becomes the priority, the 'number one' in the mother's life. The mother's existing identities have to shift to be able to make space and time for this new identity as a mother, which often occupies a predominant space.

New mothers can experience a loss of a sense of identity, freedom, independence and self-centredness whilst welcoming and learning how to balance their new mother identity into their personal dimension of existence. The unique paradox in the mother's existence is being intensely bound with another being, and at the same time being a free and separate self. The ambiguity of motherhood is in the tension of experiencing both at the same time (Butterfield 2010; Arnold-Baker 2015), and making choices and taking responsibility for both existences, her child's and her own. These choices often generate feelings of rejection and acceptance, helplessness and control, vulnerability and power.

Heidegger (1962) rejects the concept of self and instead speaks of *Dasein* (literally 'there being') which is always in relation to others and the world, as *being-in-the-world*. In reference to motherhood, when a mother accepts her new life project, which includes choices and responsibility for both existences, she accepts motherhood, the transformational journey that re-shapes her personal world, her relationship with herself and her being-in-the-world as a mother.

Deurzen and Adams describe an existential view of self as 'the dynamic centre of gravity of a person's network of physical, social, personal and spiritual worlds relations and these networks are continuously reordered and rebalanced' (Deurzen and Adams 2011: 160). They argue further that the sense of true-self shifts and changes on a daily basis and adjusts to new situations through new choices and relations: 'The paradox is that we gain a resilient and coherent sense of self because of and not in spite of our ability to be different in different circumstances. In other words, we gain a sense of authority, of being the author of our own lives' (ibid.: 71). Being-in-the-world as a mother, being responsible for the other (her child), a woman becomes more mindful of her authorship of her own life. As Heidegger (1962) and Sartre (1946) pointed out, the awareness of responsibility triggers an awareness of authorship, an awareness of creating one's own destiny, encouraging one to re-evaluate one's own values, choices and feelings in more mindful, authentic modes of living. However, this authentic mode of living, this awareness of freedom and the responsibility for creating one's own life and being the author of one's own being-in-the-world create vulnerability. Garland's (2019) research demonstrates how a new mother's awareness of their freedom of choice and of responsibility and authorship of their being-in-the-world can trigger a great level of anxiety and guilt.

Deurzen and Arnold-Baker further argue that there is a part of us that wants to affirm itself and have others affirm it too, and that prompts us to conform to the norms and expectations of the 'they'. They highlight that

> If one resists the 'they' there is a risk of rejection, isolation and an anxious confrontation with one's freedom. So we attempt to relieve ourselves of

> choosing our own possibilities and play it safe – this lessens our anxiety by bringing us a tranquillity for which everything is "in the best of order" (Deurzen and Arnold-Baker 2005: 222).

Garland (2019) suggests that motherhood puts a woman in a unique position where she is challenged to become more aware of and to redefine the balance of her authentic and inauthentic modes of living. Motherhood encourages a shift in experience of self in relation to the other, when a woman learns how to put the other before the self, and thus gaining a new awareness of herself and the other. This does not mean the sacrifice of self: instead, it is the reconstruction of the sense of self through a connectedness to the child. As McMahon (1995) states, women speak of a 'lost sense of self' using the language of traditional motherhood ideology to symbolise the process of self-change, which they purport can be very challenging but at the same time deeply meaningful.

The transition to motherhood is in essence a process through which a woman learns to relate to her child as number one, through acceptance of the responsibility for her child's being-in-the-world. This process challenges her to re-evaluate and re-assess not just what type of mother she wants to be or what values are important for her to pass on to her child, but essentially to ascertain what it means for her to be a good mother. Furthermore, and possibly as a result of this transitional process, a woman also becomes more responsible for herself, learning to live in a more mindful, authentic mode, embodying her values of 'good mothering'. She embraces an acceptance of her own limitations and gains an openness towards her own possibilities of being-in-the-world as a mother. Therefore, motherhood facilitates a transformation of personal qualities, such as becoming less self-centred, more patient, grounded, self-confident and compassionate towards oneself and others. McMahon demonstrates how becoming a mother leads to a sense of profound personal change by occasioning both the transformation of self and the rediscovery of self. As McMahon also highlights, "the self-transformation of motherhood was at once both integrating and liberating: The new and the old were born and reborn" (McMahon 1995: 151).

Furthermore, this self-transformation and self-recognition indicate self-evaluation. Weaver and Ussher (1997) assert that the loss of ego experienced through mothering is a sacred calling to self-realisation and evolution. Garland (2019) also points out that mothers do not describe self-sacrifice and self-loss, but self-reconstruction, enhancement and empowerment. Thus, the experience of empowerment and self-transformation in motherhood is a progressive, not regressive process, a flourishing from inside, not outside, that accords with the philosophy of spirituality (Athan and Miller 2013).

This shows that the mother-child relationship ushers in a profound shift in ethical conduct, as mothers become protectors of their changed values and priorities. Compassion (love, kindness, generosity, altruism) also develops as a source of great strength, which re-aligns them with a deep experience of relatedness and connectedness to their children and others, transitioning them from self-centredness to self-giving (see also Vieten et al. 2006; Athan and Miller 2013; Garland 2019).

Responsibility in the Spiritual Dimension

According to Deurzen (1984), the Spiritual (*Uberwelt*) dimension of existence centres on how we make sense of the world through our values, beliefs, priorities and how we create meaning in our lives. Garland (2019) believes the mother-child relationship can be seen as being beyond the relational field and points to a spiritual connection that nurtures not only the growth of the child but also the transformational growth of the mother. As McMahon emphasises, mothering encompasses an essence-making process and therefore inverts the conventional idea that 'mothers produce children' and looks instead at how 'children produce mothers' (McMahon 1995: 4). Athan and Miller, in their study on how motherhood provides an opportunity to learn spiritual values, compare motherly unconditional love, the 'essential foundation for love-of-other' to the quality of divine love experienced in 'the presence of the Creative principle (God)' (Athan and Miller 2013: 229). Mothers often admit that the love they experience towards their children has no limits and cannot be compared to any other feeling of love they have experienced previously (Garland 2019). Athan and Miller demonstrate how "Mothers insisted that they could not adequately capture the 'profoundness', or 'purity', with words" (Athan and Miller 2013: 231).

Through accepting responsibility for their children's well-being, mothers willingly prioritise their children's needs and move away from self-centredness. This is described as a central spiritual value, or self-transcendence. Athan & Miller term this "turning away from the self as the main source of significance" (ibid.: 233), whilst McNeill argues that spiritual development and growth are facilitated by "free participation in the breaking down of an immature, prideful self" (McNeill 1998: 334).

The above description of a mother-child relationship is reflected in the core concept defined as spiritual transformation. As the result of an act of willingly accepting the responsibility and commitment for their children, mothers experience profound and empowering spiritual growth. The developing relationship between the mother and child promotes transpersonal or mystical qualities. This prompts mothers to experience their authentic self, a heightened sense of understanding of the sacred, a greater awareness of unconditional love within their own being, and a shift in perception regarding the self in relation to the world. This can usefully be thought of as the search for transcendent meaning in life (see also Athan and Miller 2013; Matsu-Pissot 1998).

Arnold-Baker (2015) describes how the road to motherhood is paved with 'the unknown' in all four dimensions of existence, and as Athan and Miller (2013) argue, the not knowing paradoxically allows mothers to be open to their experiences. If spirituality 'connotes the self's existential search for ultimate meaning through an individualised understanding of the sacred, then mothers indeed have lived this out fully' (Wink and Dillon 2002: 73). Arnold-Baker (2015) further underlines how motherhood generates a sense of purpose, a direction in mothers' lives and a new sense of meaning. Mothers often report finding new meaning through their relationships with their children, seeing their new meaning and purpose through helping their children grow and develop.

Accepting responsibility for the other which comes from the relationship between mother and child prompts women towards a deep appreciation of the complex nature of life. From this new position, mothers can demonstrate a striking ability to face and embrace ambiguity, ambivalence, the unknown and form an ability to create meaning and purpose out of their experiences of being mothers.

Yalom uses 'purpose' in life and 'meaning' in life as interchangeable and also aligns the terms 'significance' and 'importance' in his discussion of meaning. He describes a personal meaning (or 'terrestrial meaning') that '…embraces purpose: one who possesses a sense of meaning experiences life as having some purpose of function to be fulfilled, some overriding goal or goals to which to apply oneself' (Yalom 1980: 237). He highlights the important questions we ask ourselves, such as 'How shall we live?' 'How does one proceed to construct one's own meaning – a meaning sturdy enough to support one's life?' (ibid.: 346). On the transitional journey to motherhood, mothers are confronted with questions such as, 'how do I mother?' 'How shall I live as a mother?' Examining the changes to mother's 'being-in-the-world' (across all four dimension of existence) clearly shows how they discover meaning in life through transcending their own self-interests and striving towards taking responsibility for their children's well-being and development.

Self-transcendence is the fundamental feature of Frankl's approach to the question of meaning. What a human being needs, Frankl says, 'is not a tensionless state but rather a striving and struggling for some goal worthy of him' (Frankl 1978: 38). Mothers prioritise their children's needs and well-being willingly, which echoes Frankl's belief that the striving implies freely orienting oneself towards something outside of the self.

Many researchers have shown how traditionally and continuously through history and across cultures, women are expected to sacrifice their needs and interests to motherhood, to play nurturing roles at home and in society. However, these days women have been brought up in a society with many possibilities and choices in life. Choosing motherhood as their meaning and purpose in life is only one of many choices available for women. Even though being a mother is not always a planned happening, accepting motherhood is a choice. This argument highlights the ambivalence in mothers' free choices in accepting the responsibility of motherhood, the responsibility that intensifies their awareness of existential givens and intensifies the (existential) anxiety awakened by their more mindful and authentic ways of being-in-the-world.

As Yalom points out, "one's making of meaning is anxiety soothing, it comes into being to relieve the anxiety that comes from facing a life and a world without an ordained, comforting structure" (Yalom 1980: 463). He argues that meaning gives birth to values, to some set of guidelines or principles which help us decide how to live. We need values to navigate our way of behaving in an approval-disapproval hierarchy, to help us to exist in society or belong to a group. Even though, from an existential point of view, we create ourselves through free choice, we search for some sort of structure, rules or guidance on which we can base those decisions and choices. According to Yalom, "Our human needs for overall perceptual frameworks and for a system of values on which to base our actions together constitute the 'pure' reasons that we search for meaning in life" (ibid.: 465).

Arnold-Baker (2015) speaks of how motherhood has always been seen as a life-changing experience. On every level of the mother's existence, there is a change and therefore there is no place in which the mother feels settled and at home. Addressing this side of the argument, when finding themselves in this new, unknown world of motherhood, new mothers need to find meaning and purpose to be able to re-evaluate and rebuild their value system, to comfort their anxiety and to make sense of their experiences, choices and responsibilities and to be at home in their being-in-the-world as a mother.

Addressing the complex nature of the transition to motherhood from existential perspectives reveals a bio-psycho-socio-spiritual transformation in the new mothers' being-in-the-world. Women are shaken out of their known being-in-the-world and confronted with the naked reality of the existential givens across all four dimensions of existence (Prinds et al. 2013), where they undergo physical, social, psychological and spiritual changes in life (Tammentie 2003; Stadlen 2004; Vick and Hafting 2012; Prinds 2013; Athan and Miller 2013; Arnold-Baker 2015; Garland 2019).

However, the transition to motherhood can be seen as a positive shock, that, through pain and possibilities, women are offered a personal turning point, the opportunity for a new life. It could allow women to transition from the forgetfulness mode of living into a mindfulness mode of living, or an authentic mode of living (Heidegger 1962). For new mothers it is the period that generates existential considerations regarding the meaning of new life circumstances and context, which is the essential motivation for living (Frankl 1978; Yalom 1980; Jacobsen 2007). Through reflecting on their choices and responsibility mothers are confronted by existential anxiety and guilt, as they are inextricably linked and this leads mothers to gain an understanding of how they are living in a social web and an appreciation of what authentic and mindful living means. This could help by steering new mothers away from self-criticism and self-blame towards a new opening and understanding of themselves and their position in the world, through an acceptance of their responsibility and through awareness of their agency in their choices.

References

Adams, L. G., Harper, A. J., Johnson, E. P., & Cobia, D. C. (2006). New Mothers and Sexual Intimacy: An Existential Framework for Counselling. *The Family Journal, 14,* 424–431.

Allen, A. T. (2006). *Feminism and Motherhood in Western Europe, 1890–1970: The Maternal Dilemma.* New York: Palgrave Macmillan.

Arendell, T. (2000). Conceiving and Investigating Motherhood: The Decade's Scholarship. *Journal of Marriage and the Family, 62,* 1192–1207.

Arnold-Baker, C. (2015). How Becoming a Mother Involves a Confrontation With Existence: An Existential-Phenomenological Exploration of the Experience of Early Motherhood. *Degree of Doctor of Counselling Psychology*, Middlesex University Repository.

Athan, A. M., & Miller, L. (2013). Motherhood as Opportunity to Learn Spiritual Values: Experiences and Insights of New Mothers. *Journal of Prenatal and Perinatal Psychology and Health, 27*(4), 220–253.

Barclays, L., Everitt, L., Rogan, F., Schmied, V., & Wyllie, A. (1997). Becoming a Mother—An Analysis of Women's Experience of Early Motherhood. *Journal of Advanced Nursing, 25,* 719–728.

Barlow, C. A., & Cairns, K. V. (1997). Mothering as a Psychological Experience: A Grounded Theory Exploration. *Canadian Journal of Counselling, 31*(3), 232–247.

Bergum, V. (1989). *Woman to Mother: A Transformation.* Westport, CT: Bergin & Garvey Publishers Inc.

Butterfield, E. (2010). 'Days and Nights of a New Mother': Existentialism in the Nursery. In S. Linott (Ed.), *Motherhood: Philosophy for Everyone.* West Sussex: Wiley-Blackwell.

Darvil, R., Skirton, H., & Farrand, P. (2008). Psychological Factors That Impact on Women's Experiences of First-time Motherhood: A Qualitative Study of the Transition. *Midwifery (2010), 26,* 357–366.

Ehrenreich, B., & English, D. (1978). *For Her Own Good: 150 Years of the Experts' Advice to Women.* New York: Anchor Books.

Frankl, V. E. (1978). *The Unheard Cry for Meaning: Psychotherapy and Humanism.* Oxford: Simon & Schuster.

Garland, V. (2019). 'Being-In-The-World' as a Mother Hermeneutic-Phenomenological Exploration of Lived Experiences of Eight New Mothers' Transition to Motherhood Within the Theoretical Frame of 'Four Dimensions of Existence'. *Degree of Doctor of Counselling Psychology*, Middlesex University Repository.

Hartley, J. (2005). *Transgressing the Skin: A Phenomenological Study Into the Transition to Motherhood.* (A thesis submitted in partial fulfillment of the requirements of Bournemouth University for the degree of Doctor of Philosophy). Bournemouth University, 1–379.

Heidegger, M. (1962 [1927]). *Being and Time* (trans. J. Macquarie & E. S. Robinson). London: Harper and Row.

Jacobsen, B. (2007). *Invitation to Existential Psychology. A Psychology for the Unique Human Being and Its Applications in Therapy.* London: John Wiley & Sons Ltd.

Jaspers, K. (1994). *Philosophy II. Existenzerhellung* (Philosophy II. Illumination of Existence). Munchen: Piper.

Leonard, V. W. (1993). Stress and Coping in the Transition to Parenthood of First-time Mothers with Career Commitments: An Interpretive Study (Doctoral dissertation, University of California, San Francisco). *Dissertation-Abstracts-International, 54*(08A), 3221.

Lintotte, S. (2011). *Motherhood—Philosophy for Everyone.* London: John Wiley & Sons.

Matsu-Pissot, C. (1998). On the Experience of Being Unconditionally Loved. *Phenomenological Inquiry in Psychology, 321–334.*

McMahon, M. (1995). *Engendering Motherhood. Identity and Self-Transformation in Women's Lives*. New York: Guilford Press.

McNeill, J. (1998). Psychotherapy and the Spiritual Journey. *Journal of Religion and Health, 37*(4), 333–344.

O'Reilly, A. (2010). Outlaw(ing) Motherhood: A Theory and Politic of Maternal Empowerment for the Twenty-First Century. *Hecate, 36*(1/2), 17–29.

Parker, R. (2005). *Torn in Two. The Experience of Maternal Ambivalence* (2nd ed.). London: Virago Press.

Price, J. (1988). *Motherhood: What It Does to Your Mind*. London: Pandora.

Prinds, C. H., Hvidt, N. C., Mogensen, O., & Buus, N. (2013). Making Existential Meaning in Transition to Motherhood—A Scoping Review. *Midwifery*. http://dx.doi.org/10.1016/j.midw.

Rich, A. (1977). *Of Woman Born: Motherhood as Experience and Institution*. London: Virago Press.

Ruzza, C. S. (2008). *A Phenomenological Inquiry into the Experience of First-time Motherhood After Age Forty*. New York: Fordham University.

Sartre, J. P. (1946). *Existentialism and Humanism* (trans. P. Maire). London: Methuen.

Sevon, E. (2009). Maternal Responsibility and Changing Relationality at the Beginning of Motherhood. *Studies in Education, Psychology and Social Research*, 365.

Smith-Pierce, S. (1994). Juggling: A Heuristic Study of First-time Midlife Mothers (Doctoral dissertation, The Union Institute). *Dissertation-Abstracts-International, 55*(04B), 1655.

Stadlen, N. (2004). *What Mothers Do. Especially When It Looks Like Nothing*. London: Piatkus Books.

Stadlen, N. (2011). *How Mothers Love*. London: Piatkus Books.

Stern, D., & Bruschweiler-Stern, N. (1998). *The Birth of a Mother: How Motherhood Changes You Forever*. New York: Basic Books.

Stern, D. N. (2004). The Motherhood Constellation: Therapeutic Approaches to Early Relational Problems. In A. J. Sameroff, S. C. McDonough, & K. L. Rosenblum (Eds.), *Treating Parent-Infant Relationship Problems: Strategies for Intervention*. New York: Guilford Press.

Tammentie, T., Paavilainen, E., Astedt-Jurki, P., & Marja-Terttu, T. (2003). Family Dynamics of Postnatally Depressed Mothers—Discrepancy Between Expectations and Reality. *Journal of Clinical Nursing, 13*, 65–74.

van Deurzen, E. (1984). Existential Therapy. In W. Dryden (Ed.), *Individual Therapy in Britain*. London: Harper and Row.

van Deurzen, E. (1997). *Everyday Mysteries: Existential Dimensions of Psychotherapy* (2nd ed.). London: Routledge.

van Deurzen, E., & Adams, M. (2011). *Skills in Existential Counselling and Psychotherapy*. London: Sage.

van Deurzen, E., & Arnold-Baker, C. (2005). *Existential Perspectives on Human Issues: A Handbook for Therapeutic Practice*. Basingstoke: Palgrave Macmillan.

Vick, K., & Hafting, M. (2012). "Smile Through It?" Keeping Up the Facade While Suffering from Postnatal Depressive Symptoms and Feelings of Loss: Findings of a Qualitative Study. *Psychology, 3,* (Special Issue), 810–881.

Vieten, C., Amorok, T., & Schlitz, M. M. (2006). I to We: The role of Consciousness Transformation in Compassion and Altruism. *Zygon*®, *41*(4), 915–932.

Weaver, J. J., & Ussher, J. M. (1997). How Motherhood Changes Life—A Discourse Analytic Study with Mothers of Young Children. *Journal of Reproductive and Infant Psychology.*, *15*(1), 51–68.

Wink, P., & Dillon, M. (2002). Spiritual Development Across the Adult Life Course: Findings From a Longitudinal Study. *Journal of Adult Development, 9*(1), 79–94.

Woollett, A., & Nicholson, P. (1998). Postpartum Experiences. In A. Walker (Ed.), *Niven, C, A* (pp. 88–106). Butterworth Heinemann: Current Issues in Infancy and Parenthood. Oxford.

Yalom, I. D. (1980). *Existential Psychotherapy*. New York: Basic Books.

5

The Existential Freedom of Mothers

Naomi Stadlen

Is there a sense in which a mother is free? She is usually described as 'tied down' or 'trapped' or even, as the novelist Rachel Cusk wrote when she became pregnant for the second time and longed for the freedom of her prematernal self, like a convict returning to her 'old cell' (Cusk 2001: 2).

Simone de Beauvoir was in no doubt. She made her point many times in *The Second Sex*.

> There is one female function that is still almost impossible to undertake in complete freedom, and that is motherhood.…Even one child is enough to entirely paralyse a woman's activity. (de Beauvoir 2011: 751–752).

What kind of activity did de Beauvoir believe was paralysed? She thought women should look far beyond motherhood to make free choices about how to live their lives—exactly as men did and, for that matter, as she was doing.

N. Stadlen (✉)
The New School of Psychotherapy and Counselling, London, UK

C. Arnold-Baker (ed.), *The Existential Crisis of Motherhood*,
https://doi.org/10.1007/978-3-030-56499-5_5

She never planned a society in which mothers were relieved of child-care. But Plato did. *The Republic*, completed in about 380 BC, discusses his vision of an ideal society. In fourth-century Athens, where he taught, women had few rights and little independence or status outside the home (see Powell 1988: 348–403). So it must have been astounding for Plato's contemporaries to read his radical declaration:

> There is therefore no function in society which is peculiar to women as women or men as men; natural abilities are similarly distributed in each sex; (Plato 1955: 209).

But don't women bear children, and isn't that a natural ability that isn't similarly distributed? Again, Plato's thinking was radical:

> Wives should be held in common by all; similarly *children* should be held in common, and no parent should know his child, or child his parent. (ibid.: 212).

Well, but surely if a mother gave birth to her baby and went on to breastfeed, the two of them *would* know one another. Plato had thought this through. The Republic was to be organised by male and female Guardians.

> They *[the Guardians]* will arrange for the suckling of the children by bringing their mothers to the *[communal]* nursery when their breasts are still full, taking every precaution to see that no mother recognises her child; if the mothers have not enough milk, they *[the Guardians]* will provide wet nurses. They will see that the mothers do not suckle children for more than a reasonable length of time, and will hand over all the sitting up at night and hard work to nurses and attendants. (ibid.: 216).

Here we can see Plato's genius. Wet-nursing was common in fourth-century Athens. The mother giving birth would not necessarily go on to breastfeed her own child. But her wet-nurse would be answerable to her. She would still know which baby was hers. Why did Plato insist that she should not? He was describing the running of an efficient and harmonious republic. Here, he wrote, there was to be no difference between 'mine' and 'not mine'. He must have noticed that once a mother got to know her baby, she would almost certainly experience the baby as 'mine'. He didn't say what would be wrong with this, but logically it would have meant that she would then have an individual commitment that might conflict with her loyalty to the communal republic. In other words, Plato saw these mothers as a risk to his ideal. He didn't have the same concern about fathers. In this respect, he seemed to see mothers as far more powerful than de Beauvoir did.

Plato's republic was to empower women in every way except as mothers. This sounds strangely modern. It also shows how perceptive Plato was. A mother who experiences her baby as 'mine' often finds that she reorientates her whole outlook. 'Everything is different', new mothers say. Or: 'My priorities changed completely'. We need to examine what mothers mean by this. It seems to be part of a new awareness that they discover.

A quick appraisal of maternal history supports de Beauvoir. Feminists have rightly exposed the crushing effect of patriarchal societies on women. They have identified many ways in which women have suffered for millennia. De Beauvoir doubted whether ordinary mothers could enjoy anything like the freedom she had chosen. She herself never became a mother. However, her younger friend Élisabeth Badinter did.

Badinter, like de Beauvoir, assumed that the interests of mother and child could not co-exist. She praised the feminists of the 1970s who had fought for women's freedom. But she thought that mothers were now, unfortunately 'receptive to the new order of the day: children first' (Badinter 2010: 30).

> Here, pregnancy signals the end of pleasure, freedom, and the carefree life of non-mothers. Like a postulant, the future mother no longer belongs to herself. (ibid.: 67).

Does a mother no longer belong to herself? Since Badinter describes it like this, perhaps it was true of her own experience. However, the American psychotherapist Daphne de Marneffe, in her book *Maternal Desire*, acknowledged that there were many ways of being a feminist. She reflected:

> At home with the children I made sacrifices, but I did not sacrifice myself. (de Marneffe 2004: 314).

She explained that when she considered a mother's economic well-being, she believed that all mothers made sacrifices. But when she thought about a mother's emotional well-being, she believed some feminists did not appreciate how much a mother brought to the care of her child 'the authentic expression of self' (ibid.: 8).

Badinter knew that some women enjoyed being mothers. But she thought that the majority were yielding to the 'relentless message'—that when they became mothers, they had to put their children's interests before their own—out of guilt (Badinter 2010: 168). So it's interesting to hear that this wasn't how de Marneffe found motherhood. She was sure there were many mothers like her.

> …the authentic desire to mother felt by a woman herself – a desire not derived from a child's need, though responsive to it; a desire not created by a social role, though potentially supported by it; rather, a desire anchored in her experience of herself as an agent, an autonomous individual person. (de Marneffe 2004: 4).

A mother's 'experience of herself as an agent': this is an important existential position. De Marneffe shows how her life most certainly belonged to herself, and how she could express her genuine tender feelings in her love for her children.

However, some people claim that the love mothers describe is triggered by their biology, or by their instincts, and that to some extent their feelings are pre-determined. The anthropologist Sarah Blaffer Hrdy had three children and, with the support of what she called 'allomothers' (a circle of reliable mothers and others who could look after her children when she was busy) taught at Harvard University and became a professor. She was a scholarly researcher into motherhood. One conclusion she reached was that, precisely because a baby was lovable, he could limit his mother's autonomy. Babies, she thought, were designed to make their mothers look after them.

> Over tens of thousands of years, any infant whose lusciousness was detectably less, also proved ever so slightly less likely to survive. Robustness, plumpness, cuteness, were not just useful physiological attributes....For, as designed by Mother Nature, the delectability of infants seduces to quite different ends. My children's deliciousness rendered *me*...to give up bodily resources, and in my own contemporary example, most importantly, time – time, time, time, right down to the last syllable of allocatable time (when I could get no allomother to substitute) – and so to subordinate my own aspirations to their desires so we could all (more or less) contentedly take our places at posterity's table. (Hrdy 1999: 536, 540).

The significant point here is that Hrdy says she lost some agency through being a mother. 'The delectability of infants seduces...' she wrote. So Hrdy attributes to infants the power to seduce, or perhaps to Mother Nature with the ultimate power to create seductive infants. Hrdy had to 'subordinate my own aspirations' not permanently but in the way that de Beauvoir and Badinter foresaw.

So do all mothers give up precious time to their infants because they are delectable and seductive? The passage sounds as though the infants need to appeal to their mothers' delectation, almost as if their survival depends on their 'deliciousness'. But all kinds of babies survive, and not all are 'delectable'. Besides, mothers often say how much they love their babies. But surely if they were seduced, or responding solely to the designs of Mother Nature, what they experience would no longer be what we recognise as love. Love implies a person who chooses to give love.

Rebecca Walker, daughter of the feminist writer Alice Walker, kept a diary during her pregnancy.

> 'Mine is the first generation of women to grow up thinking of *[having]* children as optional.' 'It's thrilling to be opening the door to a new life with Glen *[father of her unborn baby]*, but terrifying to be shutting all the other doors to all the other lives. A part of me wants to keep an escape route open...but another part says, No, this is it, you have a child to think about now, and turns away.' (Walker 2009: 45, 44).

Rebecca Walker was right: motherhood today can be a genuine choice. If a woman doesn't want children, or not yet, there are other alternatives open to her. Saying goodbye to some of these alternatives, as Walker recorded, can indeed be terrifying. A psychotherapist working with a pregnant woman is likely to hear anxieties about this. It can help the mother greatly to acknowledge her fear, before she gives birth, to a non-judgemental therapist. And even after conception, she gives up the familiar freedom of being responsible only for herself. However, freedom is never complete. We are always free in some respects, but not in others. So are mothers also free, even though not in the way that freedom is usually described?

The practice of mothering may look repetitive and routine, but most kinds of work have routine aspects. And mothering has something special going for it. It's unusual work because mothers don't have to worry about selling a product. There is no such object as a 'finished child', nor a competitive market in which to sell a high-quality child, or a bargain one. There isn't a 'finished mother' either. Mothering has no inbuilt career-ladder with assessments and promotion. There are no goal-posts and no prizes or awards. Some mothers are competitive, perhaps because they are bringing the familiar ethics of their paid work into mothering, and trying to get their children, for example, into particular schools. Competing for school places, though, is extra, not intrinsic to mothering itself.

The intrinsic part of being a mother is her relationship to her child. This relationship isn't visible and seems to be 'under the radar' of most people's idea of mothering. Nevertheless, it teaches the child about understanding other people and communicating with them. If the mother can relate even moderately well, she will enable her child to grow into someone who can communicate with us. Without a mother or a mother-substitute, it's difficult for a child to work out how to navigate the complexities of a human society.

It can be strange to work very hard as a mother, but to get so little social affirmation for it. And yet, the very invisibility of these relationships gives the mother a special kind of freedom. Such freedom can feel frightening—but then true freedom usually does. A mother is constrained by the laws of the society she lives in, by the opinions of her partner if she has one, and by the strong views of the baby himself. (I am using the male pronoun for the baby in order to distinguish baby from mother.) The true freedom that mothers discover is that there are no set rules for relating. Each mother decides her own.

Within her home, a mother creates a family. A family has to run on certain principles. These principles aren't usually pre-planned. Many decisions have to be made daily, and exhausted mothers typically find themselves 'doing' a decision, and questioning themselves about it later. These questions arise because a mother may find she isn't making the same decisions that other mothers have. Her family is unique.

My main source of information about this comes from nearly thirty years of running weekly discussion meetings for mothers. The mothers who come usually live in London though many were born abroad. Some come only once; others come for months and then return with a second baby. They are not a complete spectrum of all mothers. But conversations can be deep, touching on questions about being a mother that are universal. Paradoxically, it is by recognising these questions that mothers can develop their freedom. I have used a few typical statements here from mothers to give an idea of how some of them get there.

During pregnancy, a mother can sound confident of how she wants to be. Her baby then seems less personal. 'I'm not going to be one of those mums who only talks about babies', some women say. Or: 'I expect I'm going to miss my job'. But once a mother has shared the birth with her baby, and can now see him, everything looks different. No longer is he 'the baby'. He is a person, as real as herself.

A new mother is usually inundated with practical advice. She may have had a professional career and expected herself to be capable of fulfilling the requirements of her job. At work, there was a way to 'get it right', and this is often the assumption she brings to her role as a mother. She expects health professionals and experienced mothers to guide her. The responsibility of being the mother of a newborn can feel lonely and frightening. Most new mothers are thankful for some positive suggestions.

It's only when a new mother starts to follow a suggestion which sounds sensible that she discovers its implications in practice. Each one is embedded within the suggester's own system of values. So if she reads, for example, that a mother should feed her baby regularly by the clock, and not wait until he cries from hunger, this might sound a good idea. But in practice the baby may not be hungry at the regular time and protest at being woken from a deep sleep to feed. In that case, the baby will probably be ravenous at the 'wrong' time. If the mother keeps to the suggestion of clock-timed feeds, it means overruling her baby and teaching him to feed even when he's sleepy. If, on the other hand, she decides to go by her baby and overrule the clock, there will be other decisions that follow from this (such as her days becoming less predictable).

For a psychotherapist, it can be difficult to sit with a new mother. For weeks, she may sound completely lost and bewildered. It is helpful if the therapist can see this as the typical beginning of a journey into mothering, rather than the mother toppling down a bottomless hole. The therapist can then take on the role of joining the mother as she starts on her journey. Both mother and therapist may experience some of the freedom of walking into the unknown.

If a mother likes order and structure, the early months can feel chaotic. This, too, may be difficult for a therapist to hear. The mother of a six-week-old boy wondered:

> I keep asking myself questions. That's the hard thing. Not getting tired or being lonely. I like to live a *structured* life, and being a mother's not like that. Or is it? Am I doing everything wrong? I'm confused, and that's unlike me.

The mother of an eight-month-old boy struggled with two sides of a basic question:

> My son likes me to concentrate on him, and that's what I do. But my husband says I'm spoiling him. And I've got a nasty, niggling voice at the back of my head saying: 'Don't give him everything he asks for. You shouldn't be doing that. You're spoiling him. He'll grow into a spoilt child who thinks he should have everything he asks for.' And I think: But he's only eight months. And another bit of me thinks: Eight months doesn't seem so young any more.

We live in an argumentative society. It takes a while for a mother to decide which side of an argument is *her* side. The mother of a nine-month-old daughter finally decided:

> Why is it acceptable to leave a baby to cry? If it was your friend crying, you'd *never* just leave her. I see my daughter as a person. I try to communicate it by telling people: 'I'm holding her because that's the sort of person she's like.'

She defended her decision to many people who thought she was wrong to pick up her baby every time she cried. But the point is that she used her freedom to make her choice. The people around her might question her—but no one had the right to stop her.

It's more difficult when a mother is questioning the values of her own mother. The next mother made a significant decision when her daughter was only four months old:

> My mother was a rescuer. She'd always rescue me. Now my daughter keeps rolling onto her tummy and then she can't get back. She gets very frustrated, but I don't *rush* in. I wait a bit and then I say: 'Are you all right? Would you like me to turn you back?'

A London mother was adamant about what she valued. Her daughter was then twelve months.

> When I was born, my mother lived in the North, and she'd be in and out of her mother's house, and her mother in hers. They didn't even have to knock. But I want to be a different kind of mother. I want *distance* from my mother.

Again, this was her choice. This was her family and her home, and she had the freedom to set the rule she wanted. How she managed to enforce it, I never found out.

Other mothers struggle with the values they grew up with. Here again, a therapist can help by giving the mother space to voice the dilemma. It may seem a minor issue to a person who hasn't grown up with these particular values, but the therapist may be able to recognise the power of the grandmother's value system.

> My mother always put a clean and tidy house first. I'm trying to be different, but I keep asking myself little questions like: Should I be down on the floor playing with my son *[aged fifteen months]* or should I be unloading the dish-washer?

She decided in the end to play with her son. Once the mother has decided to create her own values, she is in a responsible position. There is a lot to learn, and it's easy to make mistakes. Mothers may take decisions on behalf of their pre-verbal children, only to discover that they were not the right ones after all. They usually feel stricken. But these may be only a small errors in an otherwise good level of understanding. A therapist may help the mother to learn from them, and to put them into perspective.

> My son *[aged eight months]* would never lie down and let me change his nappy. I thought he was being difficult. But yesterday he had a session with the cranial osteopath, and the osteopath told me he had a bit of congestion on his chest. In his wisdom, he knew he mustn't lie down on the floor when I changed him. *[In tears]* I should have listened to him.

Once a mother has started to feel like herself in her relationship to her child, she may decide that she wants him to feel like himself too. This means that she is encouraging him to enjoy his own freedom of thought—and of course he doesn't always think what she wants him to. It may look like naughtiness or disobedience to an outsider who doesn't know the integrity of their relationship. But it's much more likely that the child is being experimental. He senses that his mother doesn't want him to obey blindly—so he doesn't.

> My son *[aged 4 years]* likes rules. He likes to know exactly what they are. But when it's just him and me, he doesn't keep them. When he's with other children, though, he's like a policeman!

With older children, mothers decide rules between children. It can be quite difficult when two mothers have different rules, as they often do, and the children see their friends doing things they aren't allowed to.

> *First mother*: My daughter *[aged three years]* has to share her things. We're a family. We share. Even if it's her birthday present, if my son *[aged four months]* wants it and she's not playing with it, I make her give it to him. Usually she doesn't mind.
>
> *Second mother*: We share too, but it gets a bit hard when it's a birthday present. Also I don't allow physical violence in our house. *[She had three children of three years, two years and two weeks.]*

Years later, the children will build on all this experience to sort out their own rules with their friends. I noticed two boys of about ten, standing in the pouring rain with a skateboard each, beside a tiny shelter which would have kept one of them dry, but not both. Did they take turns? No. They carefully placed their skateboards upright in the small dry area. Then the two of them stood out in the rain, both getting soaked. There was complete agreement between them that this was the right thing to do, though their mothers might not have been best pleased when they got home.

All these decisions and rules might sound trivial. But they matter. In the end, each set becomes a family system reflecting, at least in part, the values that the mother believes in. This may not be obvious to a therapist who decides to query a single rule. But it's important to see that each rule has its place within the family system and needs to be discussed as a part of a larger whole.

If the mother has a partner, the two may not always agree, and this can cause conflict as both may claim to have the better values for their children. These conflicts can be difficult to resolve. However, when they both agree, they can construct an extraordinary kind of freedom. In the privacy of home, they can hold values that may be the opposite of the society in which they live.

Is it only recently that mothers have discovered this freedom? Were they more restricted if we look back to earlier times? Societies founded on the ethics of Christianity gave mothers the task of teaching basic religious education to their children. So at first sight mothers might appear to be mere tools of the Church. But a closer look reveals a much less uniform picture. The researcher Martha Saxton, for example, compared several groups of early American Christian societies, and published her results in her book with the interesting title *Being Good*. She concluded:

> Motherhood provided some Puritan women with an arena within which they administered, advocated and interpreted morality....this gave the mothers an outlet for intellect, energy, and (within limits) creativity; and it provided a substantial measure of domestic moral authority as its reward. (Saxton 2003: 85).

One very individual example, from England, is Susanna Wesley (1669–1742), mother of Charles and John who founded Methodism. Her life story was one of dramatic setbacks but she was determined to be a good mother. She bore nineteen children, of whom ten survived. Susanna decided that none of the books for educating children were good enough for hers. So she wrote her own on many subjects, often individual ones for each child. She also arranged a weekly time slot, like a tutorial, to work with each. 'On Monday I talk with Molly, on Tuesday with Hetty, Wednesday with Nancy, Thursday with Jacky, Friday with Patty, Saturday with Charles'. She wanted her girls to have as good an education as her boys. Letters survive in which she wrote to one of her adult daughters, tackling complex ethical questions. She also quoted not only Christian texts but classical writers in the original Greek and Latin, such as Plutarch and Seneca, whom she would have expected her daughter to understand. So she was sensitive to the intelligence of each child and went way beyond what was expected of an average Christian mother (Wesley 1980: 170–171).

What about less educated mothers in poorer societies? There's an interesting study of village life in Russia during the revolutionary changes from Imperial to Soviet times. In *Village Mothers,* published in 2000, Professor David Ransel interviewed Russian and Tatar peasant women, most of whom were mothers. Despite the revolutionary political and social upheaval, these women 'were able to preserve areas of independent decision that allowed them a measure of personal control and an ability either to act on their inherited norms or to fashion a new set of values appropriate to their time' (Ransel 2000: 2). They relied very much on the support of one another, mothers told Ransel, and made their own decisions about their children's upbringing.

These are random examples, but they can't be unique. Being a mother implies responsibility, and it sounds as though mothers will resist state efforts to take it from them. So it seems likely that signs of the survival of tough motherly values can be found in almost any society.

If this is the case, a mother may be struggling with the social values outside her home, while also struggling to maintain her values within it. It sounds so much work. Where is her freedom? Her child will grow and start to assert himself. Will they have interests that conflict, as de Beauvoir, Badinter and even Hrdy said they would? Yes, they often do. Does that mean that a mother can no longer do what she likes whenever she likes? Yes, it does. So it might be tempting for an existential therapist to notice how a new mother is surrendering some of her autonomy. The therapist might point out that the mother could reclaim autonomy rather than yield to the will of her baby.

But wait! It's not quite like that. We are seeing the warming of an intimate relationship. The two are learning about togetherness. This isn't a power struggle. Or rather, if they have got into a battle of wills, the next step can't happen. If mothers feel tender and close to their babies, they experience freedom of an unexpected kind.

> *Mother*: I've learned so much from being a mother. I never used to be patient, but for my daughter *[aged 18 months]* I have gallons of patience. I always loved my sleep before, but for her….And I like to have 'me' time too, to wind down with a meal and sort of collect my thoughts together, but….'
>
> *Me*: So have you learned to share your life?
>
> *Mother*: Yes, I *have*, yes.

What kind of freedom does a mother have if she has to forego her 'me' time? Something starts after birth when the two are separated. The newborn is impressionable and truthful. He hasn't discovered that he can pretend. Nor has he been hurt by a previous relationship and become defensive. He is a beginner, and a very safe person for a mother to share her life with.

Relationships typically flourish when two people learn to trust one another, enjoy listening to one another, and feel alive together. Many women have been taught that they must look sexually attractive, *or* must avoid dressing to look sexually appealing to men; that they must prove their intelligence, *or* perhaps play down their intelligence not to antagonise other people. Whatever a woman is supposed to be, there is the possibility of failing. So—what a surprise to be with her baby. He is entirely pleased with her as she is. Her ordinary self is enough. He cries when he is suddenly hungry or over-stimulated. But there is no evidence that he blames her for it, though mothers sometimes interpret crying like this. More likely, he is crying *to* her, because she is the one who understands him and always seems to know how to make everything all right again.

For many mothers, life with their babies is a way to rediscover the joy of being themselves. A mother can experience freedom from all those pressures to be 'successful' in the eyes of others, and instead enjoy the freedom to be together with her child as herself—something that solitary 'me' time cannot provide. Like this, much love can flow. Daily activities turn into new pleasures.

> I *love* breastfeeding. It's such a lovely feeling, the closeness to my son *[aged two months]*. I was completely unprepared for loving him so much.
>
> I love my work, but I love being with my son *[aged seven months]* even better. We go swimming together and then – I'm in *heaven*!

Once ignited, this love seems to deepen with years. It's not only unalloyed joy, however. It can quickly turn into acute maternal anxiety if, for example, the child is ill. But the relationship continues to have wonderful moments when the two feel comfortable to be themselves with one another.

> My daughter *[aged fifteen months]* keeps smiling. She's got a lovely smile. We smile at each other a lot. I've never smiled as much as this in my entire life.
>
> I used to worry about what to do with my son *[aged fifteen months]* when my husband's away. But we have such lovely times together. We

> gaze across the table at each other – and it's like being on a date. We each find the other one more and more wonderful.

When there is more than one child, the mother is very aware of their differences and develops an individual relationship with each.

> My daughter *[two years]*and my son *[eleven months]* are so different. There are some things that my daughter knew when she was my son's age that he just doesn't get. But there are other things that he gets already that I spent ages teaching my daughter.

For a child, an individual relationship with his mother is usually important. It can be hurtful when a mother distances herself. The existential thinker Martin Buber describes being sent to his grandparents at the age of four. No one seemed to have told him that this was to be a long-term arrangement because his parents were getting divorced. The bewilderment and loneliness of this sensitive, bright little boy can hardly be imagined. 'When after another twenty years I again saw my mother', he recalled, 'who had come from a distance to visit me, my wife and my children, I could not gaze into her still astonishingly beautiful eyes without hearing from somewhere the word *"Vergegnung" [mis-meeting]* as a word spoken to me' (Buber, 1973: 18). He couldn't show more clearly how much children value genuine moments of *meeting* their mothers.

Unfortunately, there is pressure on mothers today to be in paid work, and many say they spend less time than they would like in 'meeting' their children. The mother of a fifteen-month-old daughter observed:

> Everything conspires to make you spend less time as a mother.

We need to watch the language we use. I often hear mothers say they enjoy 'playing' with their children. In my view, this word comes nowhere near the complexity of what they are really doing. No wonder some mothers complain that they don't enjoy time with their children.

Suppose women were to say instead that they were spending time with their children 'to use our existential freedom as mothers'. People would ask: 'What do you mean?' and they would have to come up with answers.

But this would surely help them to recognise that they were being true adults (not just 'playing'). It might also encourage existential thinkers and therapists to take a second look at the Simone de Beauvoir view of mothering, and to ask themselves whether there might be a different but entirely existential way of seeing mothers.

References

Badinter, E. (2010). *The Conflict* (trans. Adriana Hunter). New York: Henry Holt.

Buber, M. (1973). *Meetings*. La Salle, IL: Open Court Publishing.

Cusk, R. (2001). *A Life's Work*. London: Fourth Estate.

de Beauvoir, S. (2011). *The Second Sex* (trans. C. Borde and S. Malovany Chevallier). London: Vintage.

de Marneffe, D. (2006). *Maternal Desire* [2004]. London: Virago.

Hrdy, S. B. (1999). *Mother Nature: Natural Selection and the Female of the Species*. London: Chatto & Windus.

Plato. (1955). *Plato: The Republic* (trans. H. D. P. Lee). Harmondsworth: Penguin. Also *The Collected Dialogues of Plato*, edited by Edith Hamilton and Huntington Cairns. New York: Bollingen Foundation, 1961.

Powell, A. (1988). Citizen Women of Athens. In *Athens and Sparta*. London and New York: Routledge.

Ransel, D. L. (2000). *Village Mothers: Three Generations of Change in Russia and Tataria*. Bloomington and Indianapolis: Indiana University Press.

Saxton, M. (2003). *Being Good: Women's Moral Values in Early America*. New York: Hill and Wang.

Walker, R. (2009). *Baby Love* [2007]. London: Souvenir Press.

Wesley, C. (Ed.). (1980). *Susanna Wesley: The Complete Writings*. Oxford: Oxford University Press.

6

Engaging with Uncertainty and Unresolved Meanings During the Transition to Motherhood

Elizabeth Simmons

Introduction

What is it like for mothers when so much is shocking and new, when their relationships, their bodies and their identities are in flux? How do mothers respond when they are unsure of what to do for the best? How do they make sense of their maternal decisions in a culture where sources of both validation and criticism are always readily available, and the long-term consequences for their babies are unknowable? How do they respond to the mysteries and challenges of the new relationship with their baby? The claim that new mothers have to live with a great deal that may be difficult to make sense of is both intuitive and well evidenced. For example, research shows that mothers' prior expectations often clash with their experiences (Miller 2005; Nelson 2003). Yet the psychological impact of transition-related uncertainty is not well understood. The advantages of using an existential perspective to address this are twofold.

E. Simmons (✉)
Horizon Psychological Services & Pennine Care NHS Trust, Manchester, UK
e-mail: beth.simmons@horizon-psychological-services.co.uk

C. Arnold-Baker (ed.), *The Existential Crisis of Motherhood*,
https://doi.org/10.1007/978-3-030-56499-5_6

Firstly, the philosophy offers a base of ideas concerning the role of uncertainty in the human condition. Secondly, phenomenological principles can be used to investigate the nature of people's engagement with it. Not only is existential philosophy relevant for the understanding of the transition to motherhood, but, it is argued, new mothers have plenty to teach existential philosophers.

Existential philosophers view the sense of unease, anxiety (Kierkegaard 1843/2004) or absurdity (Camus 1955/2004) which can arise when our sense of meaningfulness is exposed as groundless, as an inescapable part of the human condition. Heidegger characterised existential insecurity as a sense of "not-being-at-home" (Heidegger 1953/2010: 183), experienced as an uncanniness against which we attempt to buffer ourselves through retreat into familiarity, predictability and safety.

Living with something which feels significant but not-understood is likely to expose one to this sense of uncanniness. Being unable to comprehend something meaningful may also render aspects of one's past, present or future uncertain, potentially bringing one into confrontation with what Sartre (1943/2003) thought of as another key feature of the human condition, one's responsibility to make decisions without being fully in control or aware of the consequences. For new mothers, the stakes are potentially heightened. For example, the full consequences of our choices are often unknowable, but new mothers find that their choices now affect another, new life, for which they are completely responsible. Life, especially new life, is fragile. So much change and upheaval might leave one feeling particularly exposed to the uncanny.

"A Narrative Analysis of New Mothers' Experiences of Not-Understanding"

The aim of this study (Simmons 2019) was to understand more about the psychological implications of uncertainty in the transition to motherhood. Specifically, it explored how new mothers negotiated the psychological situation in which something *felt significant*, yet, for a time at least, *remained unresolved*. Perhaps surprisingly, engaging with unresolved experiences turned out to be about much more than just making sense of them, and in some cases, not about sense-making at all.

This situation of unresolved significance was termed "not-understanding", and it was explored phenomenologically through a series of qualitative interviews with first-time mothers. Although there is insufficient space here to explore each of their stories of not-understanding, I am eternally grateful to all my participants for their honesty and generosity. Some explored their unresolved feelings about maternal decisions they had made, for example regarding how best to feed their babies. For others, the shock of their embodied vulnerability following pregnancy and childbirth had taken time to come to terms with, and for one participant, this was simply one of many shocking experiences that she was struggling to grasp. Others faced frustratingly ambiguous and unsatisfying social relationships in the context of their changed circumstances. For one mother, the not-understood was characterised more as surprise than shock, as she contemplated the strangeness of her experience of clarity and happiness in the context of an otherwise distressing situation. For most, not-understanding was an unsettling, anxious, in-between sort of space, with one participant memorably referring to it as "no-man's land" (Simmons 2019: 74). Many of the stories of not-understanding I heard veered between conflicting arguments, identity positions, or between notions of vulnerability and safety, confidence and incompetence, connectedness and disconnectedness.

The study employed an experiential narrative approach adapted from Critical Narrative Analysis (Langdridge 2007). Eight first-time mothers at between six and twelve months postpartum were interviewed. What follows is a flavour of the analytical dialogue between the findings and existential ideas.

Five Ways of Not-Understanding

In the psychological literature, people are said to be disturbed when they encounter an experience which does not initially fit within their existing worldview. Their responses tend to be characterised as attempts to neutralise this disturbance, for example by dismissing the information, creating new meanings or adapting existing ones so that the experience can be integrated (e.g. Park 2010; Proulx and Inzlict 2012). However, the mothers in this study engaged with their unresolved experiences, not necessarily in order to more fully understand them as an end in itself, but rather, in order to serve psychological functions such as avoidance or connection. Not-understanding was not merely characterised by confusion or a lack of settled meaning, but rather, it was *intentional and valuable in its own right*. So, when faced with something unresolved, the psychological task was not merely "what do I do with this experience?", but rather, "what do I do with this experience *in order to…*".

Experiences of not-understanding were intentional, both in the sense that they were about a not-understood *something* and in the sense that they were directed towards particular functions. The functions to which experiences of not-understanding were directed were embedded in, and constituted by, the interpretative world of each participant and their apriori understandings, including broader sociocultural expectations. This is consistent with Husserl's (1931/2012) idea that consciousness as a whole is always intentional, or about something, and always therefore relational.

Five functions, or ways of not-understanding, emerged from the analysis. Firstly, experiences of not-understanding could function as a means of avoiding feared phenomena, for example, difficult feelings that the person did not want to connect with. Secondly, not-understanding could be a way of bearing witness to something mysterious or hitherto under-acknowledged, without necessarily needing to puzzle it out. Thirdly, not-understanding was directed towards a need to understand what to do in the face of an important decision. It then also functioned as a space in which to choose how to interpret decisions that had already been made, particularly in terms of what these choices implied about maternal identity. Finally, people engaged with their not-understood experiences in order to better connect with themselves or others.

From Disconnection to Bearing Witness: Chrissy's Story

The analysis showed that some participants who appeared stuck in a state of not-understanding were actively, deliberately disconnecting themselves from aspects of their experiences. The starkest example of this was Irene, who said of multiple traumatic experiences "If I was to really get in touch with really how I feel, I think I could have a bit of a breakdown" (Simmons 2019: 73). The analysis showed that mothers had their reasons for wanting to avoid connecting with aspects of their experiences, for example, Irene feared psychological disintegration. In the following vignette, Chrissy's attempts to do the opposite, to bear witness to her own distress, initially seemed to be in conflict with her desire to protect the narratives she had created for herself and her baby.

Chrissy had experienced a physically gruelling pregnancy and post-birth complications that left her exhausted, sick, anxious, vulnerable and lacking confidence in her own decisions. She said that: "The shock when you're just left with this new baby, I found really difficult" (ibid.: 67). Her narrative was at various times a description, an expression, a bearing witness to and an attempt to justify and explain these difficulties: the intensity of the hardship she endured, of her acute experience of vulnerability and suffering, was itself shocking and difficult to grasp.

She was keen to place these difficulties in a narrative of triumph over adversity, as she emphasised how her confidence had since been restored, reporting that "I felt like I really got into my stride with it all [...] I've just really really enjoyed, kind of every minute with her" (ibid.: 115). However, the need to bear witness to her hardship was set against a tendency to minimise her difficulties, for example, through the use of incongruent laughter:

> *Chrissy*: I think that I didn't have very much time to think about a lot to be honest, 'cause if I wasn't (laughs), wasn't being sick I was at work, and if I wasn't at work it was because I was being sick, so I erm, I didn't-
> *Beth*: -You're laughing but it sounds really miserable (ibid.: 128).

My challenging of this led initially to an assertion of the narrative to which she had been using up to this point:

> "…I don't know, it was miserable, but I don't really look back on it thinking "Oh it was a miserable time" 'cause I think I think of what the outcome was. That's how I think I look back on it." (ibid.: 129)

But then she reflected further and revealed a motivation for her self-denial.

> *Chrissy*: I didn't enjoy it as I was going through it at all […] But I think you feel bad sometimes saying that, cause you don't like, I don't wanna look back on it and I don't want to say out loud "Oh, I hated it at the time", 'cause then I think some people would be like "Oh but you got a good baby at the end of it, so"… (ibid.: 129).

Reflecting further still, she comes to a deeper motive for denial of this aspect of her experience, which is concerned with protectiveness over her child: "Perhaps I wouldn't want anyone to think that I didn't enjoy my experience of, kind of growing her" (ibid.: 129).

Chrissy seemed to be saying that she had prevented herself from acknowledging or understanding the miserable aspects of her experience as a means of protecting her baby, and particularly, the story of what it was like "growing her". Stories about what motherhood is like evidently mattered a great deal to Chrissy (and other participants who expressed similar sentiments), because they were part of her child's story as well as her own, and she felt a sense of responsibility to make this a good story somehow. Not-understanding an aspect of her experience which threatened this functioned as an attempt to protect her baby and their shared narrative.

Once Chrissy was able to make her misery explicit, she stated that she was relieved and acknowledged that:

> I think that maybe there's been a bit of recognition for myself from today that it's maybe been a bit harder than I maybe give myself credit for I think, possibly. (ibid.: 67)

The meanings of hardship and preciousness associated with growing her baby now had space to coexist, and the act of bearing witness had enabled her to move beyond her experience of not-understanding.

From an existential perspective, Chrissy's story could be framed as a journey from avoidance of some aspects of her experience, to fuller, or in Heidegger's terminology, more "authentic" (Heidegger 1953/2010: 184), ownership of the totality of her experience, including the acceptance of paradoxical meanings (of hardship and preciousness). Indeed, Chrissy's story reminds us that connection with, and acceptance of, the fullest possible spectrum of our experience may be psychologically beneficial, if only adequate time and space can be found for this endeavour. Not-understanding in this sense represented a space for the tension between owned and unowned experience.

However, Chrissy's experience is also a caution against the sometimes simplistic attempt by existential theorists or their interpreters to frame authentic engagement with one's experience and choices as necessarily more desirable, and even morally superior, to inauthentic forms of engagement. There may be good reasons why authentic, full ownership of one's experience is not always the top priority. New motherhood represents a stark test of any philosophy of how to live, because injunctions must meet the test of compatibility with the imperative of doing what needs to be done to care for a newborn. As Chrissy's story shows, this may include, not just the physical care, but care for the narrative context in which the baby grows.

Another way of looking at this is to acknowledge that the mothers in this study did not always have adequate time or space to attend to their own psychological needs during the initial transition period and had to prioritise accordingly. Indeed, several participants indicated that they had temporarily avoided engaging with their unresolved experience in order to attend to the immediate practical demands of their babies. This is to be learned from rather than judged, although we can, and should, question why self-care and protection of a baby can be felt to be in conflict. We should also ask what can be done to support mothers, both during this period, and later when they may feel more able to go back and engage with those experiences that they could not fully make sense of at the time.

Not-Understanding and Maternal Decision-Making

Several of the mothers in this study were confronted with important decisions, which had to be made despite a sense that they were not sure how best to proceed. For example, Hannah and Briony had to decide how to respond when their babies would not feed, and Ellen spoke about the difficulty of taking decisions regarding issues such as weaning and sleeping routines in the face of criticism from others. Not-understanding in the midst of decision-making was a vulnerable place to inhabit, but it functioned as a space in which to sort through conflicting ideas about what was to be done for the best, in order to make a decision. This was also a space in which existential tensions concerning choice and responsibility were particularly heightened.

The sense of shock, and sometimes crisis, that these situations invoked was driven by the mothers' newfound sense that they were now responsible for the care and protection of a defenceless baby whose well-being was overwhelmingly important to them. These high stakes rendered their inexperience and uncertainty about what to do for the best particularly threatening, and added to their sense of vulnerability. In some cases, expert advice was available, but it was not necessarily always reliable, consistent or appropriate to their individual circumstances. Thus, they were faced with the full, isolating weight of responsibility for their choices: they could ask for advice but were faced with Sartre's (1947/2007) observation that "to choose an adviser is nevertheless to commit oneself by that choice" (Sartre 1947/2007: 33).

The unpleasant shock was exacerbated because these were situations over which they had expected to wield more control, for example by choosing whether to breastfeed and how long to continue. When their babies did not fall into line with these prior expectations and choices, and when they found that they did not automatically know what to do for the best despite enormous efforts of care and attention, the mothers found themselves cut off from culturally available narratives of competent parenting.

The Hermeneutic Choice

Once decisions had been made, some participants faced another decision which I will call a "hermeneutic choice". Even where participants were broadly happy with the decisions they had made, something was left unresolved for them. This was the need to choose a version of the truth—about how to frame what had happened, what the consequences were likely to be for their babies, and what that meant for their identities as mothers. When faced with a choice of how to make sense of an experience, some interpretations threatened participants' identity or values, extending the experience of vulnerability.

Engagement with maternal decisions, both in the midst of them and later when making a hermeneutic choice, was an uncomfortable place marked by isolation and tensions. However, it was also the process through which they found their own voice and values, and by which they came to more fully own their choices as mothers.

Not-Understanding and Decision-Making: Briony's Story

Briony's story detailed the earlier-than-planned ending of her breastfeeding relationship with her baby. Her experience of not-understanding concerned "Questioning whether I'm doing the right thing, whether I'm doing the best thing for my child" (Simmons 2019: 96). She described, step by step, her anxiety and distress as breastfeeding became increasingly difficult, despite her attempts to implement the advice of various professionals. Her baby started to lose weight. He was admitted to hospital at just ten days old, and she found herself torn between a desire to continue to breastfeed because she had been convinced, in line with official advice, that this was best for him, and the temptation to switch to formula to address the crisis of weight loss. She was terrified of losing him, and asked for the doctor's advice, which was frustratingly ambiguous. She decided to offer him formula whilst attempting to continue to express milk. The crisis was averted and he began to put on weight, but her milk supply went into decline and the breastfeeding relationship ended much sooner than planned.

Not-understanding in the midst of decision-making was for Briony a space in which the loneliness and weight of her new responsibility, and her vulnerability in her new role as a mother was brought home to her:

> I suppose the decisions feel more monumental, ah, initially because there is another life involved, and also because, they're so fragile, and the situation is so fraught I suppose at the beginning because, you feel very fragile you feel very little. (ibid.: 80)

Having made her decision to use formula, Briony later grappled with what was left over as unresolved for her—her hermeneutic choice. She struggled to come to an understanding about why breastfeeding had failed, and what failure implied for herself and her relationship with her son:

> I think what's been difficult for me in my mind in coming to terms with it has been this…knowing all the recommendations around breastfeeding, knowing I haven't done that for my child. But every time I go over what happened, I know that I did what was best for my child. I do know it intellectually. Accepting that fully is, is a different thing and it is a process. (ibid.: 126)

She engaged with this unresolvedness by reflectively revisiting her left-over feelings of guilt and uncertainty about the wisdom of her decisions, and re-evaluating of breastfeeding research. She also questioned whether her expectations of herself had been realistic.

An analysis of the narrative voices in Briony's story suggested that the experience of not-understanding what it meant to end breastfeeding concerned the question of her competence as a mother, including whether it could be determined in an ultimate sense, who should determine it, and how far competence could be guaranteed by love. This was her "hermeneutic choice". Her narrative pitched a version of herself as a mother who was guilty and incompetent, against a version who was loving, imperfect but good enough, having made responsible decisions at the time in good faith. Although she was more inclined towards the latter narrative, the spectre of damning judgement expressed painfully as the thought that her son might have been better off with a different mother, persisted and had to be repeatedly confronted. By setting up a narrative dialogue between these positions or voices, the notion of competence was actively renegotiated to become something more realistically obtainable. She was ultimately able to move towards a position of greater self-acceptance. Not-understanding as hermeneutic choice had constituted a space in which to negotiate the tension between expectations drawn from culturally available good mother scripts, and the reality of her experience, partly in order to recover and rework a "good mother" identity.

Briony and several other participants all indicated that they had felt let down by health professionals when advice was either deemed absent, poor, ambiguous or inappropriate to the particular situation in which they found themselves. This disappointment was painful and threw participants into not-understanding in the midst of decision-making, in some cases accompanied by anger. Suddenly, they were faced with all of the responsibility and imperative of choice, but with none of the expected experienced reassurance which might guide their decisions.

Such experiences can be viewed on one level as examples of failures of support services. For example, it is possible that with better support, Briony's baby might have been persuaded to breastfeed. However, the experience of being let down by official advice can also be seen as a step towards more authentic and confident decision-making. From an existential perspective, authenticity is not a way of being that can be adopted wholesale and permanently, but rather, is something momentarily achieved when we grasp, or own, the possibilities and limitations before us as they are, as fully as possible (Spinelli 2005). The situations where participants felt let down by professionals required them to face the groundlessness of their choices more fully, and led to a more authentically "owned" engagement with their own decision-making process, with Chrissy, for example, coming to "trust..myself and my own kind of measure on my baby" (Simmons 2019: 68).

In cases where participants found greater autonomy after wrestling with a hermeneutic choice, and where fuller, more honest connection with self/other was being sought, one can see something recognisably transcendent in the experience of not-understanding. In this sense, the findings contradict De Beauvoir's (1949/1997) suggestion that motherhood is antithetical to transcendent, independent choice-making. On the contrary, as Briony's story suggests, not-understanding in the context of new motherhood opened up opportunities for the evolution of more autonomous, authentically owned decision-making styles. Not-understanding cannot, however, be uniformly described as either a flight from, or move towards, a more honest confrontation with existential givens. For example, Irene's inability to be at home with herself was a flight from a reality which felt too threatening to face, a form of opposition to, rather than an embrace of, the existential condition which Heidegger seems to suggest with his concept of "not-being-at-home" (Heidegger 1953/2010: 183).

The shadow of potential and actual baby loss was present in a number of stories including Briony's. Anxieties about babies' vulnerability, for example checking that they were still breathing, anxieties around bonding and concerns about feeding, all had participants' acute awareness of their babies' existential fragility at heart. As well as being "about" vulnerability, this was also about a confrontation with death and loss. The limits of responsibility and competent care, and of existence itself, were brought into focus, because the intense care and concern (love) that the participants showed for their babies could not remove the possibility that they might be separated from them permanently. From an existential perspective, Briony's questioning of her own competence, and of how far this could be guaranteed by love, can also be seen as a proxy, or expression, of this existential conflict between death and love. Perhaps not-understanding was a reflection of the unresolvable nature of this conflict.

Not-Understanding in Order to Connect

The fifth and final way of not-understanding identified in the study was the sense in which not-understanding was a search for connection. Connection meant love, openness, belonging, commitment and emotional engagement, as well as relatedness to a support network.

Dinah and Frida were motivated to reconnect with social others where they had felt isolated, abandoned or rejected. This was painful, and they each became stuck in a "why" mode of engaging, like detectives trying to piece together others' motives. Connection with experiences was also a route to understanding, for example, once Frida allowed herself to feel the pain of rejection, she was able to reconnect with her own values and decide to move on from the group.

Experiences of not-understanding seemed to force participants to inhabit simultaneously disconnected and connected ways of being. In the midst of not-understanding, participants were disconnected, cut adrift from narratives about themselves and the world on which they may have previously relied, or from people to whom they wished to feel close. An awareness of some form of disconnect or barrier to connection was necessary for the appraisal that something was not-understood, and this was generally anxiety-provoking. At the same time, an attitude of openness, to new connections, new relations of meaning, and to the work of understanding itself, was required, in order to engage with this and to reach more solid ground.

Connection had particular meaning in the context of new motherhood because of the processes of attachment and bonding. Like Briony, Hannah, Frida, Grace and Irene found both pain and solace in the motivation to stay connected to their babies. For example, Briony worried that she and her son might have lost out on a bonding opportunity because of her decision to introduce formula, and this made her experience of not-understanding significant. Resolving her sense of not-understanding in part involved learning to trust the relationship and connection that she did have with her baby, and this was also true for Hannah.

Hannah's Story—Accepting Not-Understanding in Order to Connect

Hannah's son often refused to feed, even when she was sure he was hungry. As well as engaging in various attempts to understand and fix this problem, she worried about the implications of not-understanding his behaviour, since this seemed to threaten the otherwise strong connection she had with him:

> …[W]e've had an amazing relationship and we can communicate in so many ways […]But this […]we've not/I don't understand what, what's been going on for [baby], and I feel like if I'd known, I could have tried to fix it. (Simmons 2019: 91)

Her interview was a process of peeling back layers of painful thoughts and feelings prompted by her not-understanding of his feeding behaviour. She had assumed that breastfeeding her son would provide him with the best possible start, and it was something she wanted and expected to be able to do. However, her son frequently refused her offer of the breast, and later, refused much of the nutritious solid food she offered him. The refrain which was initially front and centre in this experience, was an exasperated "why?":

> I guess it just goes back to not understanding why, why are you not hungry? Why would you not just eat whatever I'm putting in front of you? You know, not knowing the answer. (ibid.: 108)

This not-understanding why triggered a range of thoughts and feelings. She was anxious at finding herself still responsible and concerned for his nutrition, but without the control she had expected to wield. She felt angry with him, which in turn prompted guilt. Beyond the anger and guilt, Hannah found that "when I think about it too much, I feel really sad" (ibid.: 108). Hannah became tearful at the point where she connected to her sense of disappointment: "it goes back to me feeling like I haven't done the right thing or that I've let [baby] down in some way I think" (ibid.: 108).

This is the not-understanding which appeared to be at the heart of the experience. When she asked "why doesn't he eat?" or "why don't I understand why he doesn't eat?", to some extent that was a diversion from the pain, an attempt to convert it into something over which she might have some control, if she could only find the answer. However, since her son could not provide these answers, she found herself stuck.

It was only when she allowed herself to connect with the pain of the experience of not-understanding her son, that she was able to re-establish some peace of mind. There might still have been sadness, there was still no answer to the question "why?", but there was a sense of relief, and an opening up to new possibilities of interpretation. Once she had acknowledged this pain, for example, she started to be more open to the ways in which she did feel connected to her son, and she found a narrative which contained his behaviour sufficiently—instead of being incomprehensible, her son was "just really, really headstrong". She said that "you have to accept that they are their own people, with their own personalities" (ibid.: 72–73).

Not-understanding her son, feeling disconnected from him, was Hannah's source of pain. The mode of engagement with not-understanding in which she searched for answers to "why?" was partly an attempt to manage and vanquish this pain, but it was ultimately unsuccessful. It was the mode of engagement characterised by connection, that is, openness to and acceptance of, this pain, which was her route to greater understanding, openness towards and acceptance of her son.

Hannah's desire to ensure that her son fed properly was clearly motivated by concern for his well-being and not simply a desire to control him. Had his refusal to eat led to dangerous weight loss, it is probable that the question "why?" would have become far more urgent. However, Hannah's sadness and anxiety at feeling disconnected from her son, and later her willingness to accept her inability not just to understand, but to control, his behaviour, can also be seen as involving a move away from viewing him as someone to be objectively shaped by her parenting decisions to someone whose being was to be accepted and enjoyed. The distinction between these two forms of relating echoes Buber's distinction between "I-it" and "I-thou". Buber (1937/2010) suggested that "All real living is meeting" (Buber 1937/2010: 17), and that people are seeking a form of openness in their relationships with others (I-thou), which inevitably alternates with, but is ultimately more enriching than, the form of relating which sees people in terms of their function (I-It). For Buber, I-thou relating constitutes an openness to the others' presence, not delineating what or who or why they are, but recognising, accepting and affirming *that* they are present with us in a shared existence.

Buber's theory speaks to the satisfaction and peace of mind that seems to have accompanied this change in emphasis for Hannah. It is possible that participants' experiences of disconnection may have included the experienced absence, not simply of others, but of particular qualities of relating to them, such as the I-thou mode described by Buber. If, as Buber suggests, this mode of relating has the capacity to affirm us in our existence, then the absence or loss of it may plausibly be the cause of anxiety sufficient to motivate participants to negotiate the no-man's land of not-understanding.

Conclusions

This study demonstrated that people are motivated to wade into the no-man's land of not-understanding by a range of existing desires, beliefs and anxieties which shape the ways in which people then choose to engage (or choose to avoid engaging) with their experiences. I started out wanting to find out, *what do mothers do with their experiences of not-understanding*? But a better formulation of the question turned out to be "*what do mothers do with not-understanding in order to..?*", for example, in order to avoid feared phenomena, bear witness to a mysterious or under-acknowledged aspect of their experience, negotiate a decision's meaning or re-establish connection with others. Not-understanding emerged as an active, valuable psychological space in its own right.

The findings demonstrate that existential concerns may well be part of the context of a host of very practical, immediate choices which are part of the territory of new motherhood, and that these may be rendered more significant, more fragile, more disturbing and/or more potentially meaningful, as a result. In the murky no-man's land of not-understanding, tensions between existential conditions such as uncertainty, groundlessness, thrown-ness, responsibility and freedom were exacerbated, and this called for a response. The different functions of not-understanding outlined here represent different frameworks for possible actions to take in the face of the uncertainty created by these tensions. It is probable that more examples would emerge if the study was repeated with different samples.

Living with an unresolved situation was often disorientating, anxiety-provoking and lonely, but it was also, from an existential perspective, a particularly potent and valuable space, because it was the space where participants discovered what it was that they valued, and had to take a stand amidst the anxiety and uncertainty of the situation. Briony, Chrissy and Hannah all demonstrated this by coming to own their maternal decisions more fully.

Living with uncertainty and unresolved experiences may be a common part of new motherhood, contributing to the sense that this is a vulnerable time. The mothers were often prepared to engage with their not-understood experiences despite the risk that to do so would make them more vulnerable, and this demonstrated courage. For Tillich (2000), courage is an act of affirmation which he characterises as an openness to:

> ...The experience of the power of being which is present even in the face of the most radical manifestation of non-being. If one says that in the experience vitality resists despair, one must add that vitality in man is proportional to intentionality. (Tillich 2000: 177)

For Tillich, courage is seen as a way of responding to the conditions of uncertainty, freedom and death in such a way that affirms existence. Existential theory tends to prioritise the individual's existence. However, the mothers in this study had to affirm, not just their own existence and vitality, but that of their babies. This preparedness to stand in the no-mans' land of not-understanding in order to protect one's child is not directly addressed in existential theory. Further study of maternal courage has the potential to challenge assumptions about the fluidity of the existential conditions that shape our being, when we temporarily take over responsibility for another's being.

Reviewing the more culturally influential theories about motherhood and attachment, one finds biological explanations of behaviour, assumptions about mothers acting on instinct and expectations about what happens naturally and what can be expected of babies in general. However, the sense of live human struggle, of reaching through not-understanding in order to better connect with their babies, which was evident in participants' stories, is missing in much of the literature.

New mothers might benefit if, instead of being told what to do by often conflicting sources of authority, they were prepared for the necessity of having to sometimes parent in uncertain circumstances, where there is not always an obvious "best thing to do". Had the need for sustained, active, engaged struggle in which difficult choices might have to be made been more predominant in these participants' expectations of motherhood, and if engagement with not-understood experiences was reframed as potentially courageous and valuable, it is plausible that some of the distress and anxiety associated with their not-understood experiences could have been mitigated.

Perspectives such as Tillich's offer the possibility of re-evaluating the idea of struggling in uncertainty, and this is a potential source of validation for mothers' efforts, repudiating the idea that competence is linked to always knowing what to do. It may be that greater acknowledgement of the struggle to make sense (or in some cases, the choice to refrain from sense-making) has the potential to affirm us in our common humanity, and this is the essential therapeutic activity from an existential perspective.

References

Buber, M. (1937/2010). *I and Thou* (R. G. Smith, Trans.). London: Continuum.

Camus, A. (1955/2004). The Myth of Sisyphus (J. O'Brien, Trans.). In G. Marino (Ed.), *Basic Writings of Existentialism* (pp. 489–494). New York: Modern Library.

De Beauvoir, S. (1949/1997). *The Second Sex* (H. M. Parshley, Trans.). London: Random House.

Heidegger, M. (1953/2010). *Being and Time.* (J. Stambaugh, Trans.). Albany, NY: University of New York Press.

Husserl, E. (1931/2012). *Ideas: General Introduction to Pure Phenomenology* (W. R. Boyce Gibson, Trans.). London: Routledge.

Kierkegaard, S. (1843/2004). Fear and Trembling (H. V. Hong & E. H. Hong, Trans.). In G. Marino (Ed.), *Basic Writings of Existentialism* (pp. 7–40). New York: Modern Library.

Langdridge, D. (2007). *Phenomenological Psychology: Theory, Research and Method*. Harlow: Pearson.

Miller, T. (2005). *Making Sense of Motherhood: A Narrative Approach*. Cambridge: Cambridge University Press.

Nelson, A. M. (2003). Transition to Motherhood. *Journal of Obstetric, Gynecologic and Nonatal Nursing, 32*(4), 465–477. https://doi.org/10.1177/0884217503255199.

Park, C. L. (2010). Making Sense of the Meaning Literature: An Integrative Review of Meaning Making and Its Effects on Adjustment to Stressful Life Events. *Psychological Bulletin, 136,* 257–301. https://doi.org/10.1037/a0018301.

Proulx, T., & Inzlicht, M. (2012). The Five "A"s of Meaning Maintenance: Finding Meaning in the Theories of Sense-Making. *Psychological Inquiry, 23*(4), 317–335. https://doi.org/10.1080/1047840X.2012.702372.

Sartre, J. P. (1943/2003). *Being and Nothingness* (H. E. Barnes, Trans.). Oxon: Routledge.

Sartre, J. P. (1947/2007). *Existentialism Is A Humanism* (C. Macomber, Trans.). New Haven: Yale University Press.

Simmons, E. (2019) *A Narrative Analysis of New Mothers' Experiences of Not-Understanding*. Unpublished doctoral thesis, University of Middlesex, UK. Available on request from Middlesex University Research Repository.

Spinelli, E. (2005). *The Interpreted World: An Introduction to Phenomenological Psychology* (2nd ed.). London: Sage.

Tillich, P. (2000). *The Courage to Be*. New Haven: Yale University Press.

Part II

Maternal Mental Health Crisis: Understanding Maternal Mental Health from an Existential Perspective

7

Through the Lens of Trauma: The Experience of Mothering a Very Premature Infant in the First Year After Hospital Discharge

Romy Shulman

Introduction: *Through the Lens of Trauma*

Trauma cannot be easily defined. It depends greatly on the individual's subjective experience rather than on objective facts. Different people may respond differently to similar traumatic events, with some people becoming psychologically traumatised, whilst others do not. However, the experience of trauma, whether considered great or small, can affect or change our responses from there on (Beck 2004; Sluiter 2013).

Birth trauma is described by Beck as:

> an event occurring during the labour and delivery process that involves actual or threatened serious injury or death to the mother or her infant. The birthing woman experiences intense fear, loss of control, helplessness and horror. (Beck 2004: 28)

R. Shulman (✉)
London, UK

C. Arnold-Baker (ed.), *The Existential Crisis of Motherhood*,
https://doi.org/10.1007/978-3-030-56499-5_7

A woman who gives birth prematurely experiences some or all of these elements which according to this definition can be understood as trauma.

Hoffman and Vallejos refer to Tom Greening's concept of 'existential shattering' to offer an understanding of trauma from an existential perspective (as cited in Hoffman and Vallejos 2019). They explain that "Existential shattering is the sudden and unexpected dismantling, or shattering, of one's self-conception and worldview as a consequence of an event or process that the individual has experienced" (Hoffman and Vallejos 2019). This is also true for mothers of very premature babies who face a sudden and unexpected change to their expectations of childbirth and becoming a mother.

Using these two points of reference as a foundation, it can be understood that a very premature birth can affect the way a mother views every aspect of her experience in the first year of her premature baby's life and beyond (Sluiter 2013). It can be said that she may experience her first year of mothering through the lens of trauma.

Exploring this distinct experience of becoming a mother to a very premature baby through the lens of trauma can help us to better understand these mothers' individual experiences, which in turn will help us to determine the support that should be provided in these circumstances. Acknowledgement of the traumatic experience through the correct professional channels could help the mother digest her personal experience, whilst assisting her to adjust to motherhood. This in turn could help with her attachment and relationship to her baby (Beck 2004; Beck et al. 2013; Sluiter 2013).

In an effort to explore this phenomenon, I carried out research to investigate how 8 women experienced mothering their very premature baby in the first year after hospital discharge. This study gained insight into each mother's personal and individual experience of this journey, and what this experience meant for them. The study showed that the experience of a very premature birth and subsequent NICU hospitalisation affected the experience of mothering these infants in the first year after hospital discharge and reflected how the emotional repercussions of a very premature birth influence the way that the mothering relationship and the mother's identity evolve slowly and tentatively over the months to follow. Whilst the research includes a broad view of the overall experience in the first year after hospital, for the purposes of this chapter I will focus on the development of the mothering identity and the evolvement of the bonding process during this period.

The Second Set of Horror

> I think um, cos I think this sort of, for the parents of babies that are in hospital that's a whole set of horror and all the rest of it, and but there's then the sort of, the next set, when you're kind of ok, um, they then just leave you to it. (Shulman 2020: 88)

The period following hospital discharge is terrifying for the new mother. The participants describe it as 'the second set of horror' (ibid.: 88) or a 'whole second cycle of scared' (ibid.: 151). Having had a lot of medical support in the hospital, the practical mothering role had been somewhat suspended. The news of their baby's discharge felt sudden and unexpected. During the NICU stay, parents can become overwhelmed by a sea of conflicting emotions and may also find it difficult to engage with the hope of bringing a healthy baby home. In the light of this, it makes sense that my participants felt shocked and surreal about the news that they were finally taking their baby home.

Heidegger emphasises that as human beings we are thrown into situations in life that we did not choose and cannot change (Heidegger and Stambaugh 1996). With the sudden announcement of discharge, the mothers felt as if they had been suddenly thrown into a mothering role that they were completely unprepared for and lacked the skills to fulfil. The relief of going home was therefore mixed with feelings of inadequacy and fear.

It can be argued that this experience may be no different from other new mothers of full-term babies. Research by Arnold-Baker (2015) has shown that new mothers of full-term babies also experience a complex transition to motherhood, and that they too feel unskilled and unused to looking after a baby. However, mothers of very premature babies relate their fears to their traumatic experience and a difficulty to suddenly adjust to trusting that their baby could function without life support machinery and hospital intervention. Therefore, even though there was a common element amongst full-term and preterm mothers in adjusting to a new experience that requires a new set of skills, the premature mother's experience is rooted within the trauma of the early birth which sets it apart from the concerns of full-term mothers and results in an intensified mothering response.

After weeks of supervised parenting on the NICU, the mothers felt as if they had no mothering instinct of their own to draw on. The quote below describes Heather's experience of hearing her baby cry for the first time and conveys how she felt in shock and completely unequipped to comfort her baby:

> She was crying and I was quite shocked and like, 'oooh how I settle her? I remember that vividly, really clear in my mind that night because it was like, 'oh, wow. What do I do? My baby's crying! Why is she crying? What's this?' (Shulman 2020: 92)

Anita had a similar experience as she explained:

> When she used to cry and she just needed me I didn't feel that need… to you know like… it was like what do I do now? How do I deal with this? Right she is crying and all of a sudden going into this blind panic. (ibid.: 92)

This highlights the emotional distance felt between mother and child. The initial trauma of the early birth experience and hospitalisation influenced the way that these women related to being a mother and mothering their baby throughout the first year.

Keeping the Baby Alive

The first few months of mothering a very premature baby at home were generally described as focused on keeping the baby alive. All the mothers described feeling an intense fear that their baby might die. The repercussions of the precarious start were not over. The babies would stop breathing for seconds at a time launching the mothers into survival mode—poised and ready to resuscitate their babies. These fears were based on realistic medical concerns related to premature birth; however, the phenomenological nature of my study also highlighted the emotional element of this fear.

After facing the reality of the possible death of their child for a prolonged period of time, and in an effort of self-preservation, mothers prepared themselves for the worst outcome. They internalised the mortality of their baby and faced the realistic possibility of its death. Once engaged in this process, it became difficult for the mothers to forget their baby's mortality, even once they were grown and healthy. As Vicky shared:

> And then of course there's kind of, you've nearly lost him so you're just kind of waiting, to make sure that you're actually gonna keep him. (ibid.: 156)

The mothers struggled to develop a trust in their baby's resilience and their ability to survive out in the world unaided. From an existential perspective, one could argue that we are always living in the space between life and death. However, although death is possible for any person at any time, it would be difficult to engage fully with life if we focused on our mortality all the time. As Jaspers explains: 'In our day-to-day lives we often evade them, by closing our eyes and living as if they did not exist. We forget that we must die, forget our guilt, and forget that we are at the mercy of chance' (Jaspers 1951: 20).

A mother of a very premature baby is plunged into engagement with all of these phenomena immediately after giving birth. After coming face to face with this reality, it became difficult for the mothers to suddenly forget about their baby's mortality invoking a sense of impending death bringing constant fear and anxiety. Facing this limitation also reminds them of their own mortality which introduces another layer of fear and anxiety. The mother suddenly realises that she is unable to control her body or her baby's body which can introduce feelings of helplessness and subordination to the limitations of existence. Arnold-Baker's (2015) research with full-term mothers draws similar conclusions suggesting that during the initial stages of motherhood 'a window of awareness opens up for the mother and she sees existence in its raw state' leading her to question her existence and her purpose in life (Arnold-Baker 2015: 207).

Moreover, the research suggests that the trauma of the overall experience brought on a generalised worry and anxiety that they don't remember being present before. Facing the sudden trauma of early birth introduces the harsh reality of our mortality and highlights the unpredictable nature of life, as Emmy Van Deurzen states: "When life is not taken for granted, existential anxiety is experienced" (van Deurzen 2012: 48). In light of this theory, it makes sense that after the trauma of premature birth, mothers not only experience a fear of their baby dying, but also a wider existential crisis, questioning resilience, purpose and meaning in life.

From an existential perspective, it can therefore be said that a new mother of a premature baby is faced with both ontic and ontological anxiety (Tillich 1952; van Deurzen 2012). She is faced with the tangible horror of her tiny fragile medically dependent baby which is a physically and scientifically based and measured process. Yet she is also overwhelmed by the sudden change of life as she knows it and understood how to relate to it. After this crude awakening, these mothers may find it difficult to adjust back into 'normal' living without contemplating their purpose and direction life, and indeed a purpose of life in general that can end so suddenly. These findings are also in line with Tom Greening's concept of 'existential shattering' applied by Hoffman and Vallejos (2019) as discussed earlier in the chapter. Mothers of very premature babies face the sudden and unexpected disruption of their expectations of birth and motherhood. Through their trauma, their vulnerability to existential limitations has been highlighted and their sense of safety has been dismantled. As a result, they need to create a new way of relating to the world around them and rebuild their sense of trust and safety in day-to-day life.

Feeling like a Mother Came Later

A Shock Transition

For the mothers in my study labour happened suddenly and unexpectedly. The participants had not yet mentally prepared themselves to give birth or to meet their baby. They remember being in shock and disbelief when seeing their baby for the first time. The participants did not feel able to identify as the mother of the baby they were looking at. As Angela so vividly describes:

> Like my first reaction was wow, he's amazing. He's so gorgeous. Where's his mum and dad? Uh is that me? (Shulman 2020: 172).

Whilst existing research describes mothers as being in denial of their situation, my findings do not indicate denial but rather suggest that events happened so quickly that it took time for the mothers to process and assimilate what had happened to them causing a delay in the development of their emotional response. The mothers' accounts show how a mothering identity and a connection with their baby developed slowly over time in parallel with their baby's growth and development.

Some mothers attribute their initial response to the early birth and the loss of the experience of skin-to-skin contact directly after birth. They also described their babies being 'whisked away' to receive urgent medical attention before they could see or connect with them in any way. It is also clear that the mothers were in a state of shock which perhaps added to their inability to feel for their babies. These perspectives also echo those found in existing research (Golish and Powell 2003; Beck 2004; Gunter 2010; Hall et al. 2013) where mothers are described as feeling shocked and overwhelmed and unable to link their emotional response with the situation they faced. These points are reflected in Heather's quotation below:

> I think as well there was the bonding element….that goes hand-in-hand with that sort of the birth and holding your child… so….I feel like….sort of going into motherhood and feeling like a mum was sort of a delayed

> process almost, and you know, I feel really an incredible bond with my daughter now, and I definitely feel like a mum, but I think it took a while for me to sort of sort of develop those feelings and emotions. (Shulman 2020: 121)

Over and above this sense of shock, the mothers recall having feelings of guilt and failure about the birth. They felt guilt about not having been able to carry their baby to term and felt it was their fault that their baby had to endure all this pain and hardship. They felt that they had failed in the mothering role and duty of a full-term pregnancy and protecting their baby from harm. This realisation that one is unable to control their body or her baby's body brings an awareness of her subordination to the limitations of existence, and may introduce feelings of helplessness and despair.

Merleau-Ponty's (2012) theory of embodiment supports this idea. He suggests that the body is central to how we experience life situations, and that the body will store memories of these sensory experiences that will influence our future interactions with the world around us (Merleau-Ponty 2012). The mothers' sense of guilt that their body failed to protect their baby during pregnancy can be viewed as an embodied sense of failure. This could affect their level of trust in themselves to physically take care of their baby.

Mothering on Autopilot

Mothering on autopilot was a strong theme mentioned by almost all of the mothers. It seems that this is a new theme that has not been highlighted in the existing research. In the early weeks at home, participants recall functioning in an automatic mode that felt disconnected from emotion. The mothers recall caring for their baby as following a care regime by rote rather than a spontaneous expression of love and care for the baby.

Some of the mothers considered whether the hospital environment had perhaps made the care seem more medicalised and structured, and whether feeling assessed by the hospital staff perhaps disturbed the natural evolvement of the caregiving. Others thought that perhaps the fear of the babies' fragility, and the lingering fear of potential loss made it difficult for them to allow themselves to connect emotionally to their babies, for fear that they might still lose them. This supports existing findings that the fear of losing the baby affected the ability of parents to connect with their baby on the NICU (Golish and Powell 2003; Gunter 2010; Hall et al. 2013). However, my research highlights the new point that this difficulty in connection extends beyond the NICU and well into the first year of the baby's life, and in some cases beyond. As Pam shares:

> I used to go and check on him before I went to bed to feel him, make sure he was still breathing. If he'd slept through the night I'd panic, you know, has something happened to him? (Shulman 2020: 97)

Vicky had a similar experience:

> My husband still has to go check he's breathing at night. I don't quite so much… (ibid.: 130)

Whilst existing research speaks about the overall lack of connection between mother and baby, participants in my research all expressed that the practical care came easily and automatically. The need to engage practically with the baby was immediate and held serious consequences. The mothers therefore engaged with this care whether they felt ready to or not. However, engaging with the baby emotionally was perceived as having less immediate consequences and could therefore take the necessary time to develop. Over and above this, an emotional connection would not be possible to engage by rote as by its nature this can only develop at its own pace. Vicky expressed this in the following;

> I always thought that that was kind of my job in a way. Was kind of, except that I…it felt like acting the role I think, sort of, fake it till you make it, yes? (ibid.: 122)

This primal instinctive mothering mode seemed to continue for the months following hospital discharge. It seems that it was only when milestones were reached, and normal development began to become apparent that the mothers felt safe enough to interact with their babies in a more emotional way.

Sartre's (2003) theory that existence precedes essence can provide an interesting existential perspective on this theme. The participants were thrust into mothering an early baby without any choice or warning. Through the physical process of giving birth, they suddenly and unexpectedly became mothers. The participants describe their early mothering experience as 'going through the motions', or 'being on autopilot'. If Sartre's theory is applied here, one could argue that their status as mothers can be considered as a physical state that precedes an emotional connection. The emotional connection then develops slowly over time through the mother's relationship with her baby and her response to her situation and environment. This is also supported by Merleau-Ponty's (2012) theory that the physical engagement is the initial basis for experience, with thought following on from this to make sense of what we have encountered.

Bonding in the Shadow of the Threat of Loss

The crude confrontation with the reality of human fragility, death and loss affected the mothers' ability to bond with their baby. The prolonged uncertainties throughout the first year caused bonding to be a slow developing process. Existing research looks at the difficulties of bonding in the early days and the NICU stay, reporting that mothers found it difficult to bond with their very premature babies (Ionio et al. 2017). It is not surprising, therefore, that when looking at the year following discharge mothers were still struggling to bond with their babies and bonding developed slowly.

A Different Kind of Bond: The Tiger Mother Bond

Whilst existing research highlights the difficulty in bonding, my research suggests that mothers did feel a connection with their babies, but that it was different from what they had expected to feel. The expression

'Tiger mother' used by one mother seemed an accurate description of the primal and instinctive bond that the mothers described feeling for their babies. Though it was not as gentle or emotional as they had expected, they could recognise an undeniable intense bond with their babies and a desperation to help them to survive. This seems different from accounts in the existing research that focussed more on the disconnection and inability to bond or feel anything for their baby (Golish and Powell 2003; Hall et al; 2015; Spinelli et al. 2015; Ionio et al. 2017). These mothers seemed to adapt to the unexpected mothering task and bonded in the only way they knew how to. As Angela states:

> I remember very early on I had this thing, really like a… tiger mother. Like, I dunno pride when he started feeding on his own, and encouraging him was really visceral. But I don't think that's the same as a bond or maybe it's a kind of bond? That's not the same as the kind of loving bond. I didn't know if it was more of a like a drive for him to do well and develop and succeed. (Shulman 2020: 132)

Reciprocity in the Bonding Process

Reciprocity was an important factor in the start of bonding. The mothers recalled how the long-awaited smile and social interaction from their babies marked a change in their feelings towards them and their emerging feelings of being a mother. When their babies began to respond, it was like a reward for the mothers' hard work and validation that their efforts had meaning and purpose. As Vicky noted:

> He was about 4 months old. That's a long wait isn't it… for that first smile? We were sitting in the car in the car park. I had him on my lap and he just looked at me and this look of recognition came over his face and he just grinned at me, and I thought ah, ah, maybe having a baby is not that bad after all. (ibid.: 135)

Reciprocity has not previously been highlighted in research about premature parenting as a significant point in the development of bonding or the forming of the mothering identity. This therefore sheds new light on this phenomenon. It is interesting to note that my findings are similar to those of Arnold-Baker's (2015) research looking at the transition to motherhood for full-term mothers. Arnold-Baker (2015) found that full-term mothers also valued the start of social interaction with their babies and that this reciprocity was a significant point in their developing identity as a mother.

From an existential perspective, the bonding process of the mothers in the current study can be related to Martin Buber's theory of the 'I-Thou' versus the 'I-it' relationship (Buber and Smith 2000). Buber proposes that the 'I-Thou' relationship is a wholly reciprocal relationship where both sides fully experience the other. In contrast, the 'I-It' relationship refers to a simply functional relationship between subject and an object. In the 'I-Thou' relationship, the 'I' captures the essence of the interaction and shapes the context of the relationship. Conversely, Buber suggests, when relating in an I-it relationship, that one holds back something from oneself (Buber and Smith 2000).

The mothers in the study describe the first few months as a one-sided and largely functional relationship that lacked in mutuality and enjoyment. It was during these stages that mothers remember finding it difficult to feel a bond or connection to their babies. However, when the babies began to respond and the relationship became reciprocal, the mothers were able to relate to their babies as another person and began to feel a bond developing.

Mothering in the Wake of Trauma

Rooted in the Context of the NICU

It is noticeable in every interview that all 8 mothers automatically reflected back to the NICU experience to answer many of the questions that were related to their experiences in the first year after discharge. There was a strong sense throughout the various themes that their experience could not fully be understood unless a person had been through it themselves or had been involved with the experience first-hand in a medical way. This was a valuable insight into how their first year of mothering could only be understood within the context of their original trauma. This also shows how the trauma of the early birth and hospitalisation affects mothering and life in general going forward. This may also be the reason that peer support from fellow NICU mothers as well as other mothers of premature babies was described as an invaluable source of comfort and mothers guided and supported each other along their parallel journeys.

Delayed Processing of the Trauma

All 8 mothers described how they later realised that they did not fully acknowledge the seriousness of what they had been through until weeks or months after the birth and after their hospital discharge. The mothers describe that it was during those months following discharge, where the intensity of the danger and the fear slowed down somewhat, that the severity of their experience began to set in. One mother explained that as the worry began to subside, it made space in her mind to process what she had been through. This is also reflected in Angela's quote below:

> Yeah. It was after that first year when you know sleep was pretty settled and he was just an easier happier, baby. I think we looked back at it and were like, 'it was really quite tough. How did we get through that?' (Shulman 2020: 144)

This supports existing research on full-term mothers that has shown that mothers begin to make sense of their experiences towards the end of the first year post-birth (Arnold-Baker 2015).

Reconciling Joy and Loss

My study found that during the first year after hospital discharge the mothers felt a deep sense of loss and grief that they found hard to articulate. They found it hard to justify these feelings when they felt so grateful to have brought home a healthy child. With further exploration, the mothers shared that they were grieving over important aspects such as a normal healthy birth, holding and meeting their baby at birth, and a healthy start to life for their baby. However, they began to view these as trivial in comparison with the loss and horror that they had faced in the NICU. The sense of loss remained, but it was as if they needed permission to grieve. Nicole's quote below puts these thoughts into context:

> When we were bringing him home, there was a baby next to us and the parents were saying goodbye. [...] I didn't feel like I could say 'by the way, I'm not okay either', when somebody's just lost their child next door. (ibid.: 139)

It seems that the experience left little or no room for grieving over the very real losses that they had experienced. This was compounded by the feeling that those around them who had not had the same or similar experiences could not possibly understand what they had been through. The mothers experienced others as relating to them only in the present moment, with a tiny but healthy living baby in front of them. They felt that others could not relate or understand the trauma that had preceded homecoming, and therefore perhaps found it difficult to empathise with them. It is as if the mothers felt that they needed permission to grieve. They needed acknowledgement that although the object of their loss was not physical or quantifiable, their feeling of loss was real, and they were entitled to mourn the loss of their expectations, and the hopes and dreams that they had for their pregnancy and birth. The quotes below from Pam and Heather give a rich understanding of these paradoxical emotions:

> I'm sorry I probably sounds really shallow that I'm worried about the fact that I didn't have this big bump, and my baby's alive. So I should really just be [...] don't know, yeah, makes it hard to feel deserving of help. (ibid.: 138)

> Half of me feels that I didn't get to experience pregnancy to full term. So that last third trimester, I don't know what that's like and I didn't get

> to hold my baby until she was, well, for a day, so she was 24 hours old. (ibid.: 138)

The experience of the loss varied between mothers. Angela referred to her feelings during that first year as 'a strained happiness'. The fact that her experience could not fully meet her previous hopes and expectations meant that she could not feel a complete happiness. It was a happiness with a little bit missing—a sense of loss. However, Angela was determined to enjoy her first year and to be happy. She speaks of a cognitive dissonance, whereby she ignored the sense of loss and pretended to herself that she was happy.

Nicole, however, speaks about mourning the death of the child that she imagined. She talked about all the expectations that she had for her pregnancy, the birth and her unborn child, and she describes how at the moment of birth it was as if that child had died. She could not hope or expect anything because everything became completely unknown. She lost her ability to hope for a positive outcome. As can be common when faced with existential limitations such as death and illness, her fantasy that everything would be okay in the end had been shattered. She could not conceptualise anything to bond with and was left waiting in the space of not knowing.

A mother of a very premature baby is faced with conflicting emotions such as joy, grief, gratitude and loss. The uncertainty of her baby's survival is so prominent; however, she is encouraged to bond with her baby, to develop love for it, care for it and imagine that one day it will come home. Cooper (2003) discusses the paradoxes of human nature and the fight between recognising and accepting the finitude of life, but engaging in life in the face of this reality. As Cooper (2003) suggests, the outcome of this internal clash can result in fear, anxiety and helplessness in the mother. However, Deurzen and Adams highlight that we are always aware of our future death, and our challenge is to find a meaningful way to live our lives until that point (van Deurzen and Adams 2015).

Five years on my participants have each forged their path to their mothering identity. It seems that their meaning and understanding of their early birth experience continue to unfold and they have built their unique bonds with their very prematurely born children as is warmly expressed in their quotes below:

Nicole: "He's like my best friend now and I absolutely love him" (Shulman 2020: 125).

Jennifer: "I'll never know, you know, what the alternative would have been. If she'd been put on my chest as a healthy baby and I had never been parted from her. I won't know what our bond would have been like in that situation but as far as I can tell the bond is ok […] So yeah, I feel like physical separation was sort of compensated for by just pure, you know desperation and love towards her and it all worked out all right in the end" (ibid.: 132).

Eleanor: "It's like 'you don't have to be anything!' Like, I'm just so happy he's here. I don't care if he's not a genius or you know? With this it's like; he's well, he's here, he's cute. Yay!" (ibid.: 113).

Pam: "We're all immensely proud of our children and each other's children, and what they've achieved and their milestones" (ibid.: 117).

A Permanently Changed Worldview

All the mothers reflected on how their experience of the trauma had changed their perspectives on life. Having faced human mortality, and grappled with the reality of the unpredictability of their existence, these women's approach to life had become changed forever. Each mother described this in a different way, but all felt that they could not approach life in the same way that they had before. They noticed that this separated them from friends and family who they perceived remained in a less mature, more naïve state of existence.

From an existential perspective, these mothers' entire existence and relationship with the world may be called into question (Jaspers 1951; Yalom 1980; van Deurzen 2012; Cooper 2003). This highlights the importance of the implementation of emotional support that could potentially help mothers to address these existential questions and help them to build a new way of interacting with the world around them and with their babies (Jaspers 1951; Yalom 1980; van Deurzen 2012; Cooper 2003).

The existential perspective highlights how the initial trauma and the confrontation with mortality cause an 'existential shattering' that affects the way mothers of very premature babies are able to relate to their babies, others and the world around them. However, as Hoffman and Vallejos (2019) suggest, this presents an opportunity for growth through which the mothers can recognise a changed and more mature perspective on their lives.

References

Arnold-Baker, C. (2015). *How Becoming a Mother Involves a Confrontation with Existence: An Existential-Phenomenological Exploration of the Experience of Early Motherhood* (Doctorate). Middlesex University London.

Beck, C. (2004). Birth Trauma. *Nursing Research, 53*(1), 28–35.

Beck, C., Driscoll, J., & Watson, S. (2013). *Traumatic childbirth*. Oxon: Routledge.

Buber, M., & Smith, R. (2000). *I and thou*. Scribner.

Cooper, M. (2003). *Existential Therapies*. London: Sage.

Golish, T., & Powell, K. (2003). 'Ambiguous Loss': Managing the Dialectics of Grief Associated with Premature Birth. *Journal of Social and Personal Relationships, 20*(3), 309–334.

Gunter, J. (2010). *The Preemie Primer*. Cambridge, MA: Da Capo Press.

Hall, E., Kronborg, H., Aagaard, H., & Brinchmann, B. (2013). The Journey Towards Motherhood After a Very Preterm Birth: Mothers' Experiences in Hospital and After Home-Coming. *Journal of Neonatal Nursing, 19*(3), 109–113.

Hall, S., Ryan, D., Beatty, J., & Grubbs, L. (2015). Recommendations for Peer-to-Peer Support for NICU Parents. *Journal of Perinatology, 35*(S1), S9–S13.

Heidegger, M., & Stambaugh, J. (1996). *Being and Time*. Albany: State University of New York Press.

Hoffman, L., & Vallejos, L. (2019). Existential Shattering. In *Encyclopedia of Psychology and Religion* (pp. 1–4). Cham: Springer.

Ionio, C., Lista, G., Mascheroni, E., Olivari, M., Confalonieri, E., Mastrangelo, M., et al. (2017). Premature Birth: Complexities and Difficulties in Building the Mother–Child Relationship. *Journal of Reproductive and Infant Psychology, 35*(5), 509–523.

Jaspers, K. (1951). *Way to Wisdom.* New Haven: Yale University Press.
Merleau-Ponty, M. (2012). *The Phenomenology of Perception* (D. Landes, Ed.). New York: Routledge.
Sartre, J. P. (2003). *Being and Nothingness* (S. Richmond, Trans.). Oxon: Routledge.
Shulman, R. (2020). *Using Trauma as a Lens to Explore the Experience of Mothering a Very Premature Infant in the First Year After Hospital Discharge* (Unpublished DCPsych thesis), Middlesex University, London.
Sluiter, S. (2013). *Looking Through the Trauma Lens.* Ann Arbor: Loving Healing Press.
Spinelli, M., Frigerio, A., Montali, L., Fasolo, M., Spada, M., & Mangili, G. (2015). "I Still Have Difficulties Feeling Like a Mother": The Transition to Motherhood of Preterm Infants' Mothers. *Psychology & Health*, 1–21.
Tillich, P. (1952). *The Courage to Be.* New Haven, CT: Yale University Press.
van Deurzen, E. (2012). *Existential Counselling & Psychotherapy in Practice.* London: Sage.
van Deurzen, E., & Adams, M. (2015). *Skills in Existential Counselling & Psychotherapy.* London: Sage.
Yalom, I. (1980). *Existential Psychotherapy.* USA: Basic Books.

8

Postnatal Depression: An Existential Crisis?

Miriam Donaghy

The term 'postnatal depression' (PND) is used to describe the psychological distress that a woman may experience after she has a baby. It is used both as an everyday label for any psychological difficulty experienced after childbirth and as a formal psychiatric diagnosis of a depressive illness or mood disorder.[1] Increasingly, the term 'perinatal mental health' is used to describe these difficulties instead, in recognition that they are almost as likely to begin during pregnancy as after it (Glover and O'Connor 2002), and that whilst for some women the key symptoms are low mood, for others, the distress experienced is better described as anxiety or in some cases PTSD.[2]

An interest in the mental health of new mothers is not recent (there are references that can be traced back to Hippocrates, 400 BC); however,

[1]DSM 5 uses the term 'Postpartum Depression' rather than Postnatal depression and requires onset within 4 weeks of birth.

[2]Post-Traumatic Distress Disorder.

M. Donaghy (✉)
London, UK

C. Arnold-Baker (ed.), *The Existential Crisis of Motherhood*,
https://doi.org/10.1007/978-3-030-56499-5_8

with an estimated 20% of mothers affected by perinatal mental health (PMH) problems in the UK today (Bauer et al. 2014), there is some debate over whether they have become more prevalent.[3] Throughout recent decades, the psychological struggles of new mothers were at worst ignored, and at best seen only in terms of pathology, but whilst there is now an increasing and welcomed attention on PMH[4] problems, this still tends to focus mostly on a search for causation, or on the more extreme difficulties such as puerperal psychosis, where medical intervention is usually deemed necessary.

This chapter provides a quite different perspective by considering how an existential approach allows for a reframing of those negative perinatal experiences, characterised by symptoms of depression and/or anxiety, instead of presenting them as an understandable, rather than pathological response, to the mother's new situation.[5] It also considers how the existential therapist's stance to PMH difficulties differs from other approaches, and why it has much to offer new mothers in need of support through this important life-changing transition. The chapter builds upon my earlier research of 2001 in significant ways since it is now bolstered and informed by 20 years of practice in PMH services. This gives the research a much stronger grounding in the psychological lives of women and allows for a more nuanced understanding of existential concepts.

Beginning with an exploration of key existential themes including mortality, freedom, responsibility, identity and meaning, I draw on anonymised examples and observations from my work to demonstrate that the anxiety and despair, sometimes experienced during the transition to motherhood, is best understood as a reaction to an uncovering of the human condition and the 'limits of existence' (Jaspers 1951). Thus, what is often described as 'Postnatal Depression' may instead be viewed as an 'Existential Crisis', evoked by a new awareness of human facticity (Donaghy 2001).

[3]Indeed, depression is now the most common complication of pregnancy (British Journal of Obstetrics & Gynaecology, 2011).

[4]Evidenced by inclusion of Perinatal Mental Health provision in the NHS long-term plan.

[5]Puerperal psychosis which affects only 1 in 1000 women and where medical intervention is likely to be required is not included in this discussion.

Mortality and Thrownness

That we are born and inevitably will die, and that we have limited control over our existence, have long been considered by existential philosophers (such as Kierkegaard, Heidegger, Sartre, and Merleau-Ponty) as inescapable realities of life and crucial to an understanding of what it means to be human. For many women, becoming a mother brings with it an unveiling of these realities, not least because along with birth may also come a greater awareness of death.

A link between birth and death was until recently, and in some societies still is a very real one. Indeed, a World Health Organisation report (WHO 2015) estimated that there are 303,000 deaths each year from complications related to pregnancy or childbirth.[6] Whilst it is true that in the West risks to life greatly reduced during the last century, recent research findings in the UK suggest that up to a third of women suffer symptoms of trauma after giving birth, usually arising from their fears that they or their baby were in mortal danger (Svanberg 2019). Undeniably, for some women, giving birth means a glimpse of death, a confrontation with the possibility (albeit a small one) for herself and her unborn baby that they might die.

A concern with death, or as it might be described in Existential philosophy, the threat of 'non-being', is not confined to childbirth. The new mother's sense of her mortality is evoked in another, less dramatic, but significant way, as with the birth of her baby, she creates the next generation and thus there is a feeling of moving along in the cycle of life. As de Beauvoir explains,

> …'The birth of children is the death of parents.' This projection of herself is also for the woman the foreshadowing of her death. (de Beauvoir 1953: 514)

[6]World Health Organisation 2015. In addition, for every woman who dies in childbirth, dozens more suffer injury, infection or disease. 2.7 million babies died during the first 28 days of life and 2.6 million babies were stillborn.

https://www.who.int/reproductivehealth/topics/maternal_perinatal/en/.

As well as increasing awareness of her own mortality, the birth of her baby is also likely to intensify its significance, as the responsibility of caring for a totally dependent infant brings with it a new reason to live, or rather not to die. Women who have never before worried about dying become increasingly focused on the possibility of death, and on the fear of who will be there to care for their baby if they die.

Case Illustration

> **Alice**, a 37-year-old, first-time mother from South Africa, sought help after her doctor suggested counselling. Since the birth of her son, Lucas, six months earlier, Alice had attended hospital more than 10 times, convinced that she had a fatal illness. Each new check or scan giving her an 'all clear' brought relief for a few days, only for the anxiety to begin again with a gnawing doubt that 'they might have missed something'. Initially, Alice was so focussed on her physical symptoms that she seemed unaware of any link between her health worries and becoming a mother, but her voice cracked when she talked about having no family nearby, and about how Lucas might not be found if she died whilst her husband was away on a work trip.

It is not just her own death that becomes an issue for the new mother, she is also likely to be absorbed by fears that her baby might die. Beginning in pregnancy, the mother-to-be is focused on the survival of her baby, and subject to an increasing number of antenatal checks and scans she cannot help but be aware of her unborn infant's vulnerability. The intense concern with keeping the baby alive, and the anxiety that may accompany it, doesn't stop with the birth; indeed, it is quite likely to increase once the baby has arrived. Stern calls this the 'motherhood constellation',[7] a normal process of preoccupation characterised by fears,

> that the baby will die or … that he will stop breathing; that she will unintentionally suffocate him; that he won't eat and will waste away, or

[7]A 'unique psychic organization' or way of being-in-the-world, commonly experienced by women in modern Western societies when they have babies.

> won't drink and will become dehydrated; that he will fall because she isn't sufficiently protective, and so on … (Stern 1995: 175)

In the West, adding to the potency of the new mother's imagination, well-meaning health professionals proffer leaflets about cot death and how to reduce the risk; as well as advice on the need for immunisation against fatal illnesses. Unsurprisingly, the effect is to alert the mother further to the multiple dangers and possibility of death, thus concentrating her mind on the fragility of life, and the vigilance required to ensure her infant survives (Donaghy 2001).

Case Illustration

Vanessa, a 28-year-old nursery worker, was referred because she felt unable to bond with her 3-month-old baby son. She described how she could manage the practical care, feeding, changing, bathing, but just didn't feel like she thought she ought to feel, she didn't 'love him'. In the first session, Vanessa told me, in a matter of fact way that she had given birth to a still-born baby a year earlier and had been encouraged by everyone to 'try for another one'. She had conceived again quite quickly and thought she should be happy, but instead, she found herself unable to stop thinking about the baby that had died and feeling guilty about her lack of feelings for the baby in her arms.

As well as the unexpressed grief it became clear that Vanessa was deeply troubled by an awareness of mortality which she had never previously thought about, and by the randomness of her experience. Her challenge, which she slowly and bravely managed over time, was to face her anxiety about life's 'lack of guarantees' and yet still allow herself to love her baby.

Death is not the only 'given' that the new mother becomes ever more aware of, she is also likely to be confronted with inescapable evidence of 'thrownness[8]', the impossibility of controlling her environment or what the future may bring. For some women, this begins with the physical changes to her body once she is pregnant. In addition to changing shape, her body may make new demands; crave different foods; be upset by previously unnoticed smells; feel nauseous and less energetic; and be subject to a host of new aches and pains. De Beauvoir hints at the lack of control a woman may feel as this unfolds, describing pregnancy as 'a mystery that the mother lends herself to' (De Beauvoir 1953: 514). With this growing realisation that she cannot be 'in control', the new mother's previously held perception of mastery over her world may be severely shaken.

The comforting illusion of control is not easily re-established after the birth of the baby. With huge lifestyle changes and the sense that nothing can ever be the same again, previously well-ordered lives can feel chaotic, and those who have valued a life built on routine and structure often find this a real struggle. The reorganisation required and the overwhelming unfamiliarity are felt by many mothers as traumatic and may be frightening for even those who have strong support networks to help them through it all. When something goes wrong or does not fit with the mother's expectations, such as a traumatising birth experience; a sick baby; or difficulties with breastfeeding; the experienced loss of control can be incredibly distressing.

The effect of a new or growing awareness of both mortality and thrownness that accompanies the transition to motherhood is often to heighten feelings of anxiety and even despair which may then get labelled as a mood disorder. From an existential perspective, however, such feelings are considered reasonable responses to new and disquieting experiences.

[8]Translated from Geworfenheit, it is a concept introduced by German philosopher Martin Heidegger (1889–1976) to describe humans' individual existences as 'being thrown' (geworfen) into the world.

Freedom and Responsibility

Existentialism stresses the idea that ultimately each of us is responsible for who we are and what we become; as Sartre describes it, we are free to choose (Sartre 1943). From this perspective, whilst we may have a self-concept, it is not innate, but something we construct by our own free acts. This understanding of our 'openness' and our uniquely human experience of freedom and responsibility mean that women have choices about how to behave as mothers: they must choose to respond to their babies, to nurture rather than hurt them, to stay rather than leave them. In other words, they must actively choose to be good mothers.

A mother's sense of overriding responsibility for her infant's physical safety and optimal development means that she is likely to feel a great deal is dependent on her choices and actions. For the new mother, having the freedom to choose does not ensure that all choices will be good or wise ones, and so it is understandable that the enormity of this responsibility is felt as burdensome, and for some women can feel quite terrifying (Donaghy 2001).

Case Illustration

Anna, a 29-year-old mother from Poland, found her baby Zac's dependency both suffocating and anxiety-provoking and found being left alone with him when her partner went to work almost unbearable. Zac had reflux and colic and Anna described her experience whenever he was unsettled, as completely overwhelming her.

> I just want to run away. I don't want to deal with it. It's like the responsibility is all mine and I don't want it – not because of laziness, because I don't know what to do. I just get this feeling in my stomach, it's like sheer panic.

From an existential perspective, as well as the responsibility mothers must bear for their babies, importantly, they are also responsible for themselves. However, realising that they are in charge of their own destiny, in a world that is perceived as random and ambiguous, is for many mothers acutely anxiety-provoking. Indeed, perhaps one of the most important implications of ontological freedom is what Tillich called 'moral anxiety', an experience of existential guilt for what, and who we are, and what we achieve (Tillich 1952).

The tension generated by the need to fulfil one's potential is increasingly prevalent in modern, Western society, where to an unprecedented extent women believe they can 'have it all' and suffer guilt when they inevitably struggle to meet all the expectations on them in striving to do that.

The constraints involved in taking responsibility for a baby means that for many women the transition to motherhood is experienced as a sacrifice of their own potential, evoking the 'moral anxiety' that Tillich describes as 'the anxiety of self-rejection or condemnation' (Tillich 1952: 51–52). What makes this experience surprising for many new mothers, and therefore often crisis provoking, is the paradox with the commonly held belief that 'maternity is enough in all cases to crown a woman's life' (De Beauvoir 1953: 536). From this assumption, women are thought to have a biological inclination to become mothers, which is supposed, in the end, to overcome all other basic inclinations, but as Figes, a writer on motherhood, points out,

> They undoubtedly offset the losses, but babies can never compensate for them completely. They are two entirely separate nuggets of being. (Figes 1998: 34)

Whilst awareness of this paradox may precipitate feelings of despair and anxiety for the new mother, from the existential position these feelings are understood as a sign of awakening to the 'limits of existence' (Jaspers 1951), in particular, to the nature of human freedom, and to one's own desires to be all that one can. It is also understood that for some women there may be a struggle to feel content with a clearly defined role of 'mother', and that they may instead find themselves grappling with their need to make their own choices, take responsibility and fulfil their own potential.

Case Illustration

Gina, an Oxbridge science graduate, sought help with her low mood and anxiety after her second child. Gina found the yearning for a sense of achievement, and her inability to do anything about it a real struggle. She described how she found it difficult, especially when her husband and her friends talked about courses they were doing, or promotions and new opportunities in their work, to not feel like she was being left behind, 'stagnating'. Contributing to her depressed mood since having her second baby was the thought that she wasn't doing anything for herself or to improve herself. She said,

> I know it's mad when I'm so exhausted from not sleeping and I can't even concentrate to read a newspaper, but I keep thinking I should be doing something, a diploma or something. I know I'm not coping at the moment, but I keep thinking, (laughing) maybe I could get up earlier.

Identity and Meaning

There is an undeniable link between our sense of identity, or who we believe ourselves to be, and our emotional well-being. Having a clear sense of self enables clarity of direction and purpose which can bring with it a feeling of security.

From an existential perspective, however, as explored in the discussion on freedom, there is no essential self, only the one we construct through what we associate with, commit to, or concentrate on (van Deurzen 1998: 40). Thus, with all the changes that occur to what has constituted her sense of self before having a baby, there is for many women a sense of being deconstructed by the transition to motherhood, of no longer knowing who she is (Donaghy 2001).

Further, for existentialists, the body does not merely 'belong' to the self, it is understood as integral to the self, and thus it is inevitable, that the radical changes that occur through the process of being pregnant and giving birth, provoke a questioning of identity. The sense of transformation brought about by the physical changes that occur with pregnancy, labour, and breastfeeding, are however only the beginning. Indeed, for some new mothers there is a perception that all continuity on which their identity depended has gone, nothing will ever quite be the same again.

With the status of non-mother annihilated, the transition to motherhood forces a woman to construct herself anew, to make decisions about who she wants to be. As well as reconciling her new identity against her former self-construct, she is also likely to compare herself with role models, especially that of her own mother; and her ideals of what a mother can or should be. Stern (1995) suggests that the process of transformation and reorganisation of the new mother's identity is not only probable, but necessary, in order that she can alter her emotional investments, her allocation of time and energy, and her activities.

It is not surprising that for many women, this is an unsettling process and that the transformation is not always completed smoothly or easily. Indeed, initially, the mother's experience is often one of shock and disbelief as she struggles to come to terms with her new life and a new sense of self. For those, experiencing trauma during the pregnancy or birth, the sense of shock can be particularly profound.

Whilst it is essential to our understanding of the new mother's sense of self, to acknowledge that many of the building blocks on which identity is constructed, changed or lost, what is also noteworthy is that much of this change is construed negatively, for example, in terms of a loss of status. This, in my experience, is often felt most keenly by professional women such as doctors, lawyers, and journalists, or those, who having worked in the corporate world, find they have swapped high status, well-paid employment for the daily grind of caring for an infant, without any opportunity for positive feedback or financial reward, or to feel that what she does and thus who she is, is worthwhile.

Case Illustration

Sara, a 39-year-old solicitor, described how elated she had felt when she discovered she was pregnant, not least because failure at whatever she set her mind to, was not in her current realm of experience. Unfortunately, the elation had very quickly changed once her baby was born. Sara struggled with breastfeeding and gave up after a couple of weeks as it made her feel like a 'milking machine'. In her first therapy session, when her baby was just 3 weeks old, and clearly angry, she said,

> I can't believe what a terrible mistake I've made. I look at other women and I just don't know how they do it. I feel like 'why didn't anyone tell me it would be like this?'. It's so boring, so relentless, I just can't bear it.

As with any transition, becoming a mother is experienced by some as fulfilling, and a positive change, whilst for others there is frustration and a sense of being overwhelmed by demands with which they feel unable to cope. Indeed, it is another paradox of becoming a mother, that the hugely important purpose of nurturing a new life, caring for a dependent baby, is for some accompanied by a sense of losing one's sense of self and one's sense of meaning in life (Donaghy 2001).

Although having a baby is usually thought of as the archetypal 'happy event', a sense of loss is paradoxically prominent in many women's accounts of becoming a mother. Nicolson cites many losses including a feeling of lost femininity or sexual attraction; as well as a loss of intimacy with her partner; the loss of occupational identity, and with it, commonly, a loss of independence (Nicolson 1998: 93). Indeed, for the majority of new mothers that I have worked with, there has been at least some element of grieving for the 'lost self' and the autonomy that as a childless woman, they both enjoyed and took for granted. Further, admitting to negative thoughts and feelings, which contradict the concept of the 'happy event', often feels deeply shameful and so there is a reluctance to speak about it, and thus a sense of being trapped with the secret of their 'real' experience and with feelings of despair, or what Tillich (1952) describes as 'spiritual anxiety'.

Case Illustration

> **Kate**, an attractive 32-year-old hairdresser, who had always taken great pride in her appearance had been hospitalised early in her pregnancy, requiring intravenous steroid injections for severe vomiting. Kate attended counselling when her baby was 3 months old. She felt deeply miserable at her post-pregnancy body and desperate to get back to the regular gym sessions she'd attended for many years. 'I have just never looked like this. I'm a mess', she said (through angry tears).
>
> > I don't have time to do anything. As soon as I put her down she just cries. Some days I can't even get in the shower until Matt comes home.

Along with all the changes and accompanying losses, having a baby may also have an impact on values, which are frequently reassessed as the new mother looks at the bigger picture of her actions and attitudes with a child in mind. An existential perspective expects, indeed anticipates this shift, understanding that the past, or rather our view of it, is not set but is constantly revised, and thus, after having a baby our beliefs and even memories may be altered with an inevitable impact for what is held to be important.

Case Illustration

> **Ramesh:** A re-evaluation of beliefs and values was central in Ramesh's experience of becoming a mother. After the birth of her second baby, Ramesh, a 25-year-old woman from India found herself unhappily living with her in-laws, whom she felt to be critical and disapproving. Her health visitor had noticed her low mood and referred her for counselling. Ramesh had previously accepted her role in the family, where she had very little status and was expected to do all the cooking and cleaning for an extended family of 9, but now she found herself fluctuating between days when she was very tearful and others when she would pull out clumps of her own hair, turning her anger against herself. Ramesh spoke of her disappointment in having another daughter, and also of how she knew her husband was disappointed too. As the sessions progressed, she reflected on her own painful experience of being a girl where she had felt

> less important than her brothers, and at times she questioned the cultural values which previously she had always accepted. For Ramesh, becoming a mother had shaken her identity. Focussing on what she wanted for her daughters meant also choosing what she wanted for herself, and in so doing, defining who she now believed herself to be.

According to the seminal existential thinker, Merleau-Ponty, 'We confer upon history its significance, but not without it putting that significance forward itself' (Merleau-Ponty 1968a: 450). In other words, the context of the situation one is in when reviewing the past influences one's interpretation of it. A common example of such reinterpretation is how a woman's perceptions of her own mother may undergo a major shift after she gives birth. Indeed, it appears to be the case that even when her own mother is no longer alive, the relationship they had is very much re-examined. For some mothers, the experience of having a baby appears to have a positive impact on that relationship, as based on a new appreciation and need for support, they are brought closer together. For others, however, difficulties that were not present before or at least that were not previously acknowledged or recognised may emerge.

Case Illustration

> **Amanda,** a teacher, came for counselling, feeling anxious and depressed when her son was 9 months old. Having initially stated that she had experienced a happy childhood, as the sessions unfolded a different picture emerged. Amanda talked of her mother's withholding nature, the lack of warmth and frequent harsh punishment, and as she did so, she began to question the reality of what she had until then held to be true. There was a lot for Amanda to unpick but she was motivated by her wish to be the best mother she could be for her son. Her desire to mother differently meant reassessing the relationship she had with her own mother, which was painful and also challenging for Amanda's sense of whom she had believed herself to be.

It is perhaps of little surprise that for many women along with the 'crisis of identity' evoked by so much change and loss, there may also be a related crisis of meaning. The meanings that one attaches to one's beliefs, and values, are often altered dramatically during the transition to motherhood so that what was previously valued and provided motivation is no longer available or relevant. This in itself can be an unsettling experience. However, potentially more disturbing still for the mother's equilibrium is how having a baby may influence or even negate her sense of 'Meaning in life' (Donaghy 2001).

Meaning is a key concern in existential philosophy, considered in particular by Sartre (1938, 1946) and Camus (1942), who have grappled with how to have meaning in a world which is, apparently absurd,[9] and by Frankl (1946, 1967), for whom, the importance of meaning is that it enables us to bear the 'tragic triad of human existence' pain, guilt and death (Frankl 1967: 61). According to Frankl, the need for meaning 'is inherent in being human, and therefore indispensable to mental well-being' (ibid.: 19). Indeed, Frankl saw a lack of purpose as commonly at the root of problems such as depression and anxiety, and thus continually emphasised the importance of having goals, in order to escape the void of meaninglessness that may evolve in their absence.

I have observed in my work that some new mothers experience a sense of giving up on fulfilling their potential, no longer feeling able to pursue personal goals. The repercussions of this are that it often creates a vacuum of meaning, with some women feeling that beyond their role of mother they have no purpose.

A loss of purpose may occur for another, quite different reason for those who, in giving birth gain a longed-for baby, and achieve their cherished ambition, with the result that there often follows a sense of 'what now?' For many women, having a child is a goal they have aspired to for as long as they can remember, so once achieved there is a loss of what served as their motivating drive. This is felt particularly where women have had to overcome additional obstacles in order to either become pregnant, in cases of infertility, or to have a live baby when there have been previous miscarriages or stillbirths.

[9]The idea that our thrownness and eventual death makes the world meaningless.

Case Illustration

> **Ali,** a 39-year-old accountant, experienced four miscarriages and two rounds of IVF. Now with 6-month-old twins, Ali felt overwhelmed by their demands and was struggling to admit that being a mother wasn't what she had imagined it to be through all those years of longing. Having a shared goal with her husband of achieving what had seemed so elusive and unobtainable, had kept them close. Now that they had achieved it, what had been a joint preoccupation was gone. Worse still, with Ali feeling disillusioned about the reality of motherhood and finding it difficult to cope, their relationship had also begun to falter.
>
> > I've tried telling him how I feel, but all he says is 'It's what you wanted Ali', I feel like he's angry with me, he doesn't want to hear it, so I just shut up.

Existential Therapist Approach

As well as looking at the transition to motherhood through the lens of key existential themes, the existential therapist takes a stance that contributes to a distinct and effective approach for supporting new mothers in a number of ways.

Normalising Not Pathologising

Firstly, the mainstream view that conceptualises perinatal difficulties as pathology, seeing them in terms of deficits, defects, and abnormalities, is firmly rejected as a normative approach that results in women feeling stigmatised. It is misguided as Deurzen points out because it assumes,

> that people ought to be immune from the difficulties that their lives expose them to and that they should be able to cope at all times. We

> conclude that if they do not cope there is something wrong with them, rather than the situation. (van Deurzen 1998: 2)

An existential perspective invites us to view negative perinatal experiences in the context of the woman's life, and as 'problems in living' (Szasz 1961) that human beings may encounter. In taking this approach, unpleasant feelings and experiences, including those of anxiety and despair, are normalised, and the obstacles of shame and stigma that many women feel acutely, and which frequently prevents them either admitting the extent of their suffering or coming forward to seek help, are removed.[10]

Further, the existential position that 'there is no place for norms' (Cohn 1997: 95) means that the therapist is able to challenge the often idealised, assumptions about 'good mothering' and what should be available via maternal instinct. Such unrealistic expectations of themselves and motherhood which too often lead to feelings of failure, self-doubt and a sense that the baby's essentially normal behaviour is a manifestation of her inadequacy are common factors in many new mothers' negative postnatal experience (Donaghy 2001).

Case Illustration

> **Laura**, a 40-year-old architect, arrived with her frail-looking baby whom she explained had been 2 months premature and then wouldn't feed as he had a tongue-tie. She came because her "husband thought it would be a good idea to talk to someone." A "ditched birth-plan" and her unsuccessful attempt at breastfeeding had left Laura feeling like "a complete failure". As she repeatedly offered her baby a bottle that he didn't seem very interested in, she explained that she had been wondering if she was really cut out for being a mother.
>
>> Perhaps it would be best if I went back to work…… then he could go to a childminder who likes doing this stuff and knows how to do it properly.

---

[10]Only 15% of women with symptoms of postnatal depression actively seek or obtain medical advice (Royal College for General Practitioners 2015).

Allowing mothers to express their feelings of ambivalence, irritation, anxiety or despair with a focus on normalising these experiences can encourage the mother to re-evaluate her assumptions. In adopting an 'open attitude' and suspending prejudice around what is expected of new mothers, the existential therapist can enable a thorough and honest investigation of the mother's situation free from the fear of judgment (ibid.: 2001). Through this process, she is able to arrive at a more realistic idea of mothering, one in which difficulties are seen as inevitable, and thus she is able to acknowledge a more positive view of her own capabilities.

This was the case for Laura, whose response on her completion questionnaire to the question 'what had been most helpful?' was 'The realisation that it was ok to feel angry and disappointed and that doesn't mean I'm a bad mother'.

Subjective Not Objective

The existential philosopher Kierkegaard asserted, 'subjectivity is truth' and 'truth is subjectivity' (Kierkegaard 1844); thus, the existential therapist will choose to reject another cornerstone of most other approaches to PMH problems, namely their focus on objectivity and the search for certain, definable knowledge including a need to determine causation.

An existential approach means moving away from objective accounts and rejects the depersonalising process involved in objectification. In this way, the mother's own experience is fundamental and essential in a phenomenological investigation. Thus, what is often demoted to mere anecdote or opinion by science, a thorough understanding of each woman's story, through which some ontological characteristics may be found, becomes central (Donaghy 2001).

By moving away from 'attempts to explain the mother's predicament in relation to any theory of causation an existential therapist is free to explore and clarify the mother's current situation: to discover with the mother what it means for her. The focus then is on elucidating the mother's meaning of her experience. Does it represent sacrifice and loss, feelings about lower status, or fear of taking responsibility? Does it evoke a crisis in terms of awakening her to awareness of her own mortality?

It is only by individual exploration with the mother as we 'tease apart the strands of her resistance, her distractions, her predilections, and the essence of her wounded soul' (Kleiman 2017: 5) that we can come to understand what is at stake for her, and why becoming a mother has in her case precipitated an existential crisis (Donaghy 2001).

The existential therapist's approach, being open to, '…what needs exploring with both maximum intensity and personal involvement, and yet also with a maximum of alertness to the many angles and perspectives to the issue'. Deurzen (1998: 112), offers the opportunity to understand together, with the mother, what choices she wishes to make, where she can find meaning and how she can be supported in her struggle to find the courage to be (Donaghy 2001).

Holistic, Not Dualistic

Finally, an existential therapist opposes the inherent dualism in much of the discussion about women's struggles in the perinatal period, not just the split between mind and body but also the dichotomy of the self and world (ibid.: 2001). As Merleau-Ponty sees it, such dualism inevitably involves a distortion of our lived experience and also means a failure to appreciate the ambiguous nature of the world, and our perception of it.

As well as rejecting these dualistic splits, an existential approach means rejecting simplistic 'either-or' explanations, and theories based on a unilinear model of cause and effect because 'everything we live or think has always several meanings' (Merleau-Ponty 1968a: 169). Thus, a more ambiguous and intersubjective view of contributing factors is proposed in which the subjective experience of the individual mother is considered key, and where, 'The event of childbirth cannot be seen apart from either the individual experience or the cultural experience' (Nicolson 1998: 51).

For existentialists, this view of the interconnectedness, or intersubjective nature of the world, is an extremely important one, as can be seen in Heidegger's reference to human beings as 'Being-in-the-world' (Heidegger 1927). According to Heidegger, Dasein[11] is always in a

[11] Heidegger's term for human beings, usually translated as 'Being-There'.

world, and always in relationship, and it is not possible to consider Dasein out of this context. Indeed, this view of human existence where the individual is understood as the focal point of a network of interactions and interrelationships is one of Heidegger's most central insights.

Whilst becoming a mother is a universal experience, mothers are not a homogenous group. This is only too evident from my work at MumsAid,[12] where the mothers supported have come from Africa, Asia, Europe, Australia, China, North and South America; and have ranged in age from just 14 years old to 51. There have been some who have escaped slavery and being trafficked; and others with professional qualifications and high-status careers, some have disabilities or have disabled children, some have partners others are single, some have grown up in care and others have witnessed unspeakable traumas. For all these mothers, there are huge and fundamental differences in the stories they bring and the impact and challenges they face as mothers and it is essential to see and understand their story, their context. Indeed, it is impossible to gain a true insight into their perinatal difficulties without doing so.

Understood as one of the fundamental givens of existence, relatedness is an essential concern of existential psychotherapy. Thus, in order to make sense of the experience of transitioning to motherhood from the mother's perspective, we need to understand the intersubjective relationship of the various psychological, social, biological and temporal factors at play when women become mothers. In attempting to understand and assist the new mother in her struggle, it is important that we do not abstract her from her social and cultural framework. Instead, we must consider her in the context of her world, and in relationship (Donaghy 2001), including her relationship with her partner, her own mother and importantly her baby. What is needed is a complex and holistic view of human beings as 'bio-socio-psycho-spiritual organisms, joined to the world around us in everything we are and do' (van Deurzen 1997: 94).

[12]A charity in South East London that offers therapeutic support to pregnant and postnatal women, including teenage mothers www.mums-aid.org.

Conclusion

This chapter has suggested an alternative framework from which to consider perinatal mental health challenges, such as postnatal depression. Building upon original research which explored motherhood through the lens of an existential crisis (Donaghy 2001), it has presented the transition to motherhood with its inevitable struggles between freedom and responsibility, mortality and our thrownness into the world, identity and the universal quest for meaning, as key existential themes through which mothers might understand their experience. With this open and sensitive perspective, women need not feel pathologised, deviant or incapable but instead be supported as they experience a moment of awakening to the human condition.

The existential therapist's understanding of how and why becoming a mother may evoke an existential crisis makes her well placed to understand the anxiety and despair that this may bring, and the potential in exploring it (ibid.: 2001). Further, by normalising the mother's experience there is an opportunity for healing the shame which is so prevalent in perinatal distress, and which causes so much suffering.

Finally, but importantly, the existential therapist also offers an opportunity for the new mother to consider how she can do more than merely survive the difficulties of the transition, if she chooses to, there is the chance to come to a new understanding of life, rising to the challenges of being human as well as the new challenges that becoming a mother brings.

References

American Psychiatric Association. (2013). *Diagnostic and Statistical Manual of Mental Disorders (DSM)* (5th ed.). Arlington, VA: Author.

Bauer, A., et al. (2014). *The Costs of Perinatal Mental Health Problems*. Centre for Mental Health and the London School of Economics.

Camus, A. (1942/1975). *The Myth of Sisyphus*. Harmondsworth: Penguin.

Cohn, H. W. (1997). *Existential Thought and Psychotherapeutic Practice*. London: Sage.
de Beauvoir, S. (1953/1997). *The Second Sex*. London: Vintage Classics.
Donaghy, M. (2001). *Postnatal Depression: An Existential Crisis* (MA Dissertation). NSPC University of Sheffield.
Figes, K. (1998). *Life After Birth*. London: Little Brown.
Frankl, V. (1946/1964). *Man's Search for Meaning*. London: Hodder and Stoughton.
Frankl, V. (1967). *Psychotherapy and Existentialism*. Harmondsworth: Penguin.
Glover, V., & O'Connor, T. (2002). Effects of Antenatal Stress and Anxiety: Implications for Development and Psychiatry. *British Journal of Psychiatry, 180*(5), 389–391. https://doi.org/10.1192/bjp.180.5.389.
Greenberg, M. (1985). *The Birth of a Father*. New York: Avon Books.
Heidegger, M. (1927/1962). *Being and Time* (J. Macquarie & E. S. Robinson, Trans.). New York: Harper and Rowe.
Jaspers, K. (1951). *The Way to Wisdom*. New Haven, CT and London: Yale University Press.
Khan, L. (2015). *Falling Through the Gaps*. London: Royal College of General Practitioners and Centre for Mental Health.
Kierkegaard, S. (1844). *The Concept of Anxiety* (R. Thomte, Trans.). Princeton, NJ: Princeton University Press.
Kleiman, K. (2017). *The Art of Holding in Therapy*. London: Routledge.
Merleau-Ponty, M. (1968a). *Phenomenology of Perception* (C. Smith, Trans.). London: Routledge *&* Kegan Paul.
Merleau-Ponty, M. (1968b). *The Visible and the Invisible*. Evanston, IL: Northwestern University Press.
Nicholson, P. (1998). *Postnatal Depression: Psychology, Science, and the Transition to Motherhood*. London: Routledge.
Sartre, J. P. (1938/1962). *Nausea*. Harmondsworth: Penguin.
Sartre, J. P. (1943/1956). *Being and Nothingness: An Essay on Phenomenological Ontology* (H. Barnes, Trans.). London: Methuen.
Sartre, J. P. (1946/1957). *Existentialism and Humanism*. New York: Wisdom Library.
Stern, D. (1995). *The Motherhood Constellation: A Unified View of Parent Infant Psychotherapy*. New York: Basic Books.
Svanberg, E. (2019). *Why Birth Trauma Matters*. London: Pinter & Martin.
Szasz, T. (1961). *The Myth of Mental Illness*. New York: Harper.
Tillich, P. (1952). *The Courage to Be*. New Haven, CT: Yale University Press.
van Deurzen, E. (1997). *Everyday Mysteries*. London: Routledge.

van Deurzen, E. (1998). *Paradox and Passion in Psychotherapy: An Existential Approach to Therapy and Counselling*. Chichester: Wiley.

World Health Organisation (WHO). (2015). *Sexual and Reproductive Health*. https://www.who.int/reproductivehealth/topics/maternal_perinatal/en/.

9

Maternal Postnatal Depression: The Fathers' Experience

Farasat Sadia

Setting the Context

The birth of a child inevitably results in a major transition in the lives of new mothers and fathers. It is a major developmental event for both parents. Its effects on parents—both as individuals and as a couple—are profound and therefore it has an important impact on family life. During this period, the leading mental health complication is postnatal depression (PND) (Robertson et al. 2004), which denominates the depressive symptoms that may occur surrounding the prenatal and postnatal period. The effects of PND on the mental health of the mother are varied. However, an overlooked aspect is that fathers may also face a challenging and unfamiliar situation after childbirth, which is compounded if the mother is suffering from PND. This chapter is based on the findings of my recent research (Sadia 2020) where I aimed to find out what it is like for fathers to live with women who are experiencing PND. Their experience indicates that they also suffer a great deal alongside their partners,

F. Sadia (✉)
University of Cambridge, Cambridge, UK

C. Arnold-Baker (ed.), *The Existential Crisis of Motherhood*,
https://doi.org/10.1007/978-3-030-56499-5_9

when postnatal depression takes hold of the mother, and in their own way each father ends up learning how to live with their emotions whilst coping with the realities of life after the birth of the child. Although each family's life is a unique symphony with its own melodies, as we listen to more and more of those symphonies certain leitmotifs can be identified which denote the presence of common strands of experiences. These strands or themes demonstrate the multidimensional, often challenging and prolonged struggle that fathers have to face. It is these common strands of experience that I discuss below in more detail.

Suffering as a Couple

Life as a couple undergoes drastic changes when the mother suffers from PND and almost all these changes make it difficult for the couple to cope with the situation. This also impacts the father's ability to fulfil his role as a partner and father. Generally, clear, open and helpful communication between the couple becomes much harder during the PND phase, mostly due to time pressures and the emotional fragility of the mother. In some cases, it generates a complete breakdown of communication with some fathers trying to rationalise things that are fundamentally emotional, and which cannot be understood in a rational sense. In these moments, it feels like the fathers and mothers are not attuned with each other—as fathers try to problem solve whilst the mothers just need to be heard and accepted. Changes in the dependency the couple feel towards each other is another factor and generally, the mothers become increasingly dependent upon their partners during this time. The extent of this change in dependency varies widely though and it is quite dynamic, varying over time during the different phases of postnatal depression. The possibility that the couple cease to maintain their independence as adults because of a kind of co-dependency being created cannot be discounted here. It is quite possible that in some cases both the partners make up their minds that the changed circumstances after the birth of the baby have made it nigh on impossible for them to continue to manage their lives independently and thus, they prolong or heighten the dependency beyond their absolute need.

In most cases, the relationship between the parents sustains considerable damage during the course of postnatal depression. Most of the fathers used words like isolation, lack of affection, withdrawal, boredom, frustration and annoyance to describe how their relationships with their partners were affected. Physical and emotional intimacy became harder during the postnatal depression period as PND is detrimental to the affective, as well as the sexual side of being a couple. As the mothers become more withdrawn, wanting to be alone, there seems to be no time left for shared activities or moments together as a couple. Emotional and physical tiredness, the need for the mothers to be supported and the fathers' need for some time on their own all work against the couple.

The predominant emotion here is misery. The misery stems from and spans the issues the partners face in communicating with each other during their day-to-day lives; to the way the couple becomes more dependent on each other during PND and includes the way their relationship changes for the worse as intimacy becomes challenging. The fathers' response to the misery is multifaceted and diverse. When considering how the communication with their partners suffered, some fathers respond by accepting that this was going to remain hampered by necessity in the milieu of their changed reality; but others are not able to passively accept this change and react with anger at the loss of their cherished partner with whom they were previously able to share the burdens and joys of life. The fathers' response to this misery, which resulted from the change in the relationship dynamics, is almost universally centred on frustration and in almost all cases they strive to improve the situation despite achieving almost no success. This leads to them tolerating their transformed life with latent feelings of resentment because of perceived feelings of unfairness.

However, the fathers' response to the misery due to the loss of intimacy with their partners is different, because here most fathers accept that this aspect is going to take time to recover, and they do not feel that their needs warrant preference over the need to be responsive and empathic to their partners. Intimate partners do not merely respond to each other, but they carefully open themselves up to each other in order to gain a better understanding of the intimate-other. Buber's concept of the I-Thou relationship is relevant here: "The primary word I-Thou can be spoken only with the whole being" (Buber 1923: 11) and "True marriage always arises out of the revealing by two people of the Thou to one another. Out of this a marriage is built up by the Thou that is neither of the I's" (ibid.: 46). Thus, the intimate relationship between the partners is about openness towards each other, responding to each other, and together creating an interpersonal space between themselves which transcends each of their personal worlds and pertains to their spiritual dimension of existence. The partners relate to each other with their whole being so that, in Buber's words, they fill the heavens for one another (ibid.: 8), and in relating to each other in this manner they also address the spiritual experience of addressing the eternal Thou. Before their partners suffered from PND, the fathers are blissfully used to having an intimate I-Thou relationship with them. It is important to note, though, that this is not the only mode of relating. When they are experiencing their partners as separate human beings with their own specific characteristics cognised separately, the fleeting I-Thou relationship evaporates, and the partners become a separate "thing" for the fathers to interact with. Buber was also fully cognisant of this fact when he said that "Every Thou in the world is by its nature fated to become a thing, or continually to re-enter into the condition of things" (ibid.: 17). In an intimate relationship, the couple must be able to, at times, meet each other fully and openly in the I-Thou relationship, and be receptive to other's actions and responses, even though at other times they also need to be able to know each other in the I-It way. Unfortunately, maintaining the I-Thou way of communication and connection becomes much harder once their partners start suffering from PND. The openness and closeness needed to sustain that mode of relating disappears as PND develops. At that point, neither partner is ready to accept the genuine encounter with the other that Jaspers (1941) advocated. Jaspers believed that the opportunities for reciprocal discovery afforded by communication allows revelation of the full self (Jaspers 1941). It seems that for the couple, it becomes impossible to achieve reciprocal discovery when effective communication has become impossible. As Buber states, a life or relationship which does not know of the I-Thou mode of relating is an impoverished one, as encounter is an essential part of the human existence: "without It man cannot live. But he who lives with It alone is not a man" (Buber 1970: 34).

Living with Her PND

A big source of worry for fathers are the longer-term implications of PND on their partners. Not only do they worry about whether their partners would fully recover and return to how they had once been but also whether their relationship would survive. Fathers also worry about how long the whole process will take, whether their child would be affected in any way and whether there would be any financial implications and so on. However, having the confidence that PND is a finite illness, which would end at some point is very encouraging for the fathers. From an existential point of view, the experience here pertains to the dimension of time because the concern and worry is about the tableau in the future era in the presence of the realization that the present milieu is but evanescent and transient. It is very important for fathers to retain faith in their life as it transforms into a new reality; when the current constraints and limits no longer dictate the make-up of their family life, and they wonder what this future holds in store for them.

One of the biggest apprehensions and fears for fathers is that their wives will leave or disappear, or in quite a few cases, commit suicide. This feeling is rooted in the emotional turmoil their partners experience when they are suffering from PND. Fathers lose their trust in their partners and fear they will make an imprudent or irrational decision. This, coupled with the sadness of the mothers who are unable to find any joy in their lives at that point, and the fact that the fathers are unable to "fix" the situation, leads to fathers believing that their partners may just choose to leave or disappear. Confronting, or facing up to the existential given of death, is a very important facet brought to the fore by this apprehension felt by fathers. The risk of suicide of their partners is also a facing up to death for themselves. Death is one of the fundamental human concerns according to existential philosophy. Contemplating death lends authenticity and meaning to life (Heidegger 1927). Deurzen expresses how death is an important reminder of life and that when we come to terms with death, we start to take our lives more seriously (van Deurzen 1997). The deaths of our near and dear ones are the first portal through which death enters the realm of our consciousness. For fathers, confronting the possibility of the demise of their partner forces them to experience their fear of death head-on. The death does not need to be the actual event of their partner's demise, because as Heidegger (1927) says, human existence is a constant movement in time with the past being where we are no longer, and therefore we die a little bit each day (van Deurzen 1988). For the fathers, the fact that their partners have changed irrevocably since the birth of their child, and that their relationship has also changed tremendously, means that the partner from their past, and relationship that they had, is gone forever. Thus, the "deathly" fear that afflicts the fathers is that of irreversible loss, either through the physical death of their wives or through the loss of their partner-as-they-used-to-be and the loss of their relationship that they held close to their hearts. Different fathers of course have their own way of coping or confronting this fear. Some feel that letting themselves become paralysed or less functional is just not an option when their partners are already going through PND, so they resolve to not let themselves feel terrified or depressed. However, other fathers find it helpful to remind themselves about past experiences where they got through adversity with a positive approach, and this helps them confront their present woes with courage and determination.

It is a very hard task to be strong and to keep providing the emotional and physical support required by their partners. Stress induced by the physical effort and tiredness coupled with the stress of not being able to lean upon their partners emotionally and having to manage their emotions alone all add up to making it very challenging. The fathers cannot let themselves be vulnerable for the sake of their child who is also involved, and they are prepared to sacrifice their own needs and give precedence to the needs of their partners during this crisis period. Expressing their feelings or even making queries about general day-to-day affairs is not straightforward for the fathers. They feel their comments may be perceived in a negative light, and this ultimately generates frustration for both partners. This makes the fathers very wary of expressing their thoughts and feelings or even asking questions. They have to be careful about what they say and how they say it. They have to gather their courage and remain confident and vigilant because they feel that being vulnerable themselves means the whole family could become exposed and defenceless.

Personal Challenges

Fathers are stretched to the limit by the magnitude of the challenges facing them whilst living with partners who are suffering from PND and almost all of them feel confused and lost in the face of their problems that they had not envisaged and which they could not figure out how to tackle. Multiple sources of stress, all acting at the same time, make it very difficult to make sense of what was happening around them and how they are affected by it. Hit by the mounting demands on the physical as well as the emotional side, and with a lack of time to stop and make sense of anything, fathers start to lose hope that they can have any effect on things, which further exacerbates the emotional burden. The gist of the experience here is that fathers find themselves unable to cope with the arduous ordeal thrown their way with any degree of confidence or assurance. It starts with the fathers finding themselves ill-equipped to deal with the situation and being surprised about how horribly bad it is, thereby generating feelings of worry and confusion. From this point, a downward journey of loss starts, progressing through misery and resignation, with fathers feeling as if they are supposed to be strong enough to cope with the situation but not finding themselves being able to deal with it, resulting in them feeling miserable and sorrowful; and then finally, the journey culminates in resignation and despondency where the fathers feel completely powerless and incompetent and that all they can hope for is day-to-day survival. To them, things feel chaotic because they are not in a position to make sense of what is happening around them and they feel they do not have any control or ability to make an impact on the situation, thus exacerbating those feelings of despondency.

The experience described here is so focussed on the negative, depressive emotions that it seems like fathers lose all hope. However, this is not the full picture because fathers do find the courage to continue to support their wives and children and remain able to function socially as well as meeting the physical needs of themselves and their families. It is only in their personal, internal world that they give free reign to their emotions and thus find themselves sinking deeper and deeper without any ray of hope illuminating the way for them. In the personal world of the fathers, a sense of complete powerlessness and incompetence starts to develop. For the fathers, who in most cases are not used to these feelings, this results in new facets of their personal development coming to the fore. Much like Prinds et al. (2013) describe the mothers' experience, the Eigenwelt [personal dimension] confronts the fathers with life events that put their inner self at stake. Looking at the experiences of the fathers, crisis management helps them acquire new skills and better equips them for the future. However, at the time when they are going through the thick of it, things feel chaotic to them because they do not have the time for closer examination of their personal world to see what is happening there. All their effort and time are taken up by the other more immediate needs mostly pertaining to the other dimensions of existence, so the introspection required to become cognisant of their personal world changes is impossible. They are just aware that they are faced with a huge challenge and that they are unable to do anything that would result in its immediate improvement, hence the feelings of resignation and despondency discussed earlier. It is clear that living differently has an impact on the fathers' sense of themselves and their personal world. Where they have previously not been stretched to the extent that they run into their limits of physical and emotional endurance, the personal challenges faced when living with their wives' PND forces them into that situation. From an existential point of view, the question of how they respond at the personal level to overwhelming challenges when giving in is not an option is very important. As Deurzen has noted, hardship and difficulty are "important and necessary parts of coming to ourselves in depth" (Deurzen 2012: 7) and individuals need to become the architects of their lives rather than being passive victims of circumstances. This is exactly the personal lesson that the fathers learn, and they grow to become stronger individuals as a result of the challenges they overcome.

Emotional Roller Coaster

Fathers live through a tumultuous experience and go through the full spectrum of feelings from pride and pleasure to sadness and desperation when their wives are suffering from postnatal depression. They learn to be a new father as well as a good and supportive husband at the same time. Frustration is one of the predominant emotions during this time: mostly to do with how their partners have changed, or started to behave towards them, but also generally about not being able to see any changes for the better. The mothers fail to agree about relapses and the fathers cannot easily accept the fact that their wives seem to have been better occasionally in the past, without recovering permanently. Sometimes there is needless argumentation when their partners are trying to vent, which can be very frustrating for the fathers because they feel they haven't done anything wrong. There are hard times, and a lot of negative emotions, especially when things seem to be out of control and the fathers feel very frustrated, sometimes with their wives, sometimes with the system and sometimes with themselves.

Sadness is also a common emotion, about both lost hopes and the lost opportunities of enjoying the first year of their family life together with their young child. In particular, seeing their partner suffer extreme sadness just makes the fathers feel sad as well. Essentially, both are unable to appreciate their child's very early life well which they realise is a chance they will not get again.

At the same time, fathers also experience guilt that somehow, they are responsible, or the cause, of their wives' emotional state and postnatal depression. Or guilt for not being able to provide effective and timely physical and emotional support to their wives. In addition, in some cases, there is a feeling of unfairness which emanates from the distribution of household responsibilities, and to the way some mothers attribute the wrong reasons to the fathers' actions. There is also the feeling that they have to deal with challenging circumstances even though they have not played a big role in creating them. Delving a bit deeper, the unfairness seems to be associated with the fathers being stuck in idealised roles and feeling that they don't have the fatherhood they had wanted or expected. There seem to be preconceived notions about the father's role (mostly providing support to the mother and child and working as the breadwinner) and the mother's role (mostly taking care of the child and household work). No negotiation takes place between the partners about what their roles are going to be in the new family situation. There may be an important implication here for counsellors or therapists working with clients in similar situations, as it may potentially be helpful for clients to explore whether feelings of unfairness, frustration, the weight of expectations and other related feelings are rooted in prejudiced conceptions about the roles of fathers and mothers.

However, the fathers do take pride in their role of father. One of the main reasons for feeling proud is the perception that it is a hard role to fulfil. This naturally generates a perception about managing to overcome a very challenging situation. The fathers cling on to the hope that things are going to get better soon and that their wives would return to "normal" again, giving them the chance to relish the moments that only a young baby can provide his or her parents.

There is also joy, mostly from having achieved a certain proficiency at being a competent father and husband. However, this is not a celebrated joy that the whole family could be a part. Most of the joy is experienced in the internal, personal world of the fathers. It seems that the couple become split by the experience, with the fathers becoming self-sacrificing.

A full survey of the emotions and feelings of the fathers' inner worlds reveals a whole microcosm of experience. What we find are lots of dark clouds of frustrations, sadness, guilt and feelings of unfairness; however, all is not lost because the clouds are punctuated by rays of light where pride, joy and hope shine through. Sartre (1939) posits that frustration is the fundamental bedrock upon which all other emotions germinate and flourish. However, frustration need not be considered solely as the instrument of tragedy here because there is an ontological significance behind frustration which exposes a certain facet of our personal and social existence: the presence of frustration innately signifies the presence of a personal investment, a personal cherishing for what is desired, i.e. that which frustrates us possesses the potential to satiate us as well. Looking back at the experience of the fathers, the fact that a lot of frustration manifests itself is not surprising as it is an indicator of the degree to which the fathers are invested in the goal of keeping the family unit together and healthy, and maintaining the well-being of their wife and child as well as themselves. In a way, the emotions experienced by the fathers are signposts, marking that which they value and hold dear in their personal world. In the longer term, the emotions themselves rise and fall over time, but the values behind the emotions will always remain significant for the fathers.

Meeting Expectations

The weight of expectation, from multiple sources, affects the fathers significantly. There are three major sources of expectation: The first relates to expectations from the outside or physical world, i.e. the reality of continuing to fulfil the responsibilities of their role as the breadwinner for the family and balancing work and family life; the second relates to the personal world of the fathers where they place expectations on themselves about not letting their needs take priority and to prioritise the needs of the mother and child; and finally, the third relates to the social world where in spite of wanting to relieve their wives of a lot more responsibilities, the fathers run into situations where it is impossible to meet their wives' expectations. These factors working in unison create a situation where they are really stressed. The need for constant care and support results in some fathers even wanting to disappear for a while.

The majority of the fathers experience severe difficulties in maintaining a healthy work–life balance whilst their partners suffered from PND. In addition to the expected extra workload at home, the fathers find it difficult to concentrate at work; their thoughts distracted, and messages or phone calls from home result in interruptions and occasionally having to take extra time off work. They feel that things are piling up, even for those who have their own business. Stress induced by work deadlines, coupled with exhaustion, lack of time, lack of sleep, lack of concentration, multiple demands from colleagues and with conflicting demands from their partners all adds up to making it very hard for the fathers to meet the various expectations.

Fathers do not feel able to prioritise or put their own needs forward. They expect to be able to do this and to put themselves aside for a period of time to just let the family survive the difficult period. This is a conscious choice that they are happy to make. However, where it becomes trickier is during the recovery phase when their partners seem to have started to recover from the worst phase of PND. At this time, some fathers feel that their needs should begin to be heard, but it is hard to determine whether their partner has recovered completely or even partially. This makes it challenging for the fathers who don't know when they can start to loosen their self-imposed expectations upon themselves of putting their needs second.

It is a common feeling that the fathers do not have enough time to do everything that they need to do. This is mostly related to there being too many things left to do in the evenings after work as their partners feel unable to take care of the daily chores like making dinner, washing clothes or general cleaning whilst also taking care of the infant. Thus, the fathers face the prospect of having to choose to de-prioritise some things by necessity. Over time, it generates the feeling of a never-ending workload. Additionally, there is a worry about whether the mothers are having enough rest and support so that they would be able to take care of their child whilst the fathers are away at work.

At this time, there does not appear to be any ray of hope in the darkness for the fathers, as they cannot see how they can find a way to be successful in the face of what seem overwhelming odds. The biggest change in the personal world of the fathers is the new way in which they compel themselves to feel and behave after they became fathers. There are lots of emotions of misery because of the physical and emotional hardship, excessive responsibilities which cannot all be met, and this results in an element of despair, and vigilance in terms of not putting their own needs forward. However, fathers do not give into their feelings of despondency. The question they ask themselves is, how can I deal with the misery? and how do I prevent myself from sinking into despair and depression? When in many cases this is the hardest challenge they have had to endure in their lives. Maybe what helps these fathers is their newfound purpose, i.e. being the last line of defence for the whole family. They know that in not letting themselves sink into despair they are not only protecting themselves but also protecting their wives and children and maybe this lends a meaning to all their hardships. It gives them a reason to bear the suffering, a "why", and as Nietzsche says, for "He who has a *why* to live for can bear with almost any *how*" (Frankl 1946).

Lack of Support

During this period, the fathers suffer from a lack of support. Even though they yearn for someone they can approach for support and reassurance that they are fulfilling their role appropriately in the face of the tough and challenging circumstances, the fathers are rarely able to find people around them who can help them in this regard. Owing to the impression that their partners are the ones who have mental health issues, i.e. PND, both the professionals, as well as friends and families, focus on providing support to the mothers and thus the fathers feel ignored. But the fathers also need support and this ultimately results in feelings of frustration and disappointment, with some fathers being envious of the fact that their partners are able to access more support and help. Some fathers, however, play a role in making support difficult to access because they do not feel comfortable seeking it when they most need it. They are quite passive and do not share their difficulties or seek out help or reassurance. Although they desire support and reassurance at this time, they find it difficult to actively seek to fulfil that desire. Sharing their experience, even with close friends, is only deemed acceptable if they are confident that they are going to get useful advice, for example if they know someone who has had prior experience of similar circumstances. For some, aversion at being considered a victim is the main source of reluctance.

The experience here pertains to a deep-seated need for interaction with others and the desire for their support which the fathers crave. The behaviour of others around them strongly influences the essence of the father's experience. All their feelings and emotions occur against a backdrop of how they perceive the actions of both friends and family, as well as professionals, and how they respond to them. A variety of feelings and emotions ranging from their hope and desire for support to anger about the way they feel ignored by both professionals as well as friends and family are all present. This turns into frustration when they feel that they have been left alone in challenging circumstances which they are not able to overcome and improve themselves. Over time, some fathers start to feel desperate about the situation. From the starting point of hope and desire, the fathers' experience undergoes a progressive downward spiral through the negative emotions of jealousy, anger, frustration, despair and confusion. Whilst this paints a sorry picture of struggle and misery, the degree to which fathers crave support does vary quite significantly and not all fathers are affected by all the negative emotions with the same severity. However, generally it is clear that the perceived lack of support affects almost all the fathers negatively and they feel that they really need to draw upon social support during this critical time. This is important for their own, as well as their families, psychological well-being. As Deurzen says, we are interdependent with the world and are linked with people outside ourselves (van Deurzen 1988), this interdependency and linking with others is what the fathers desire to lean upon. Almost every individual needs to have a sense of being part of a community and being a member of a community, which provides social support and collective coping (Wong et al. 2006) so that the individual's life is enriched in proportion to the vitality and harmony of the overall community. The support of a community that the fathers crave is painfully missing in these cases. Even in a gathering of fathers whose partners are all going through PND, the men are not inclined to explore each other's experiences and therefore fail to develop a collective wisdom that may help them in collective coping.

Surviving the Situation

How to cope with their challenging situation is a major issue confronting fathers. Whilst the actual strategies and mechanisms used by the fathers to survive the tough circumstances vary according to the details of each situation and individual, some general factors are identifiable, notably the ability to bury their emotions and to adopt a more practical approach. Thinking about positive and joyful things and participating in pleasurable activities are also considered good ways to relieve the stress and recoup their ability to manage. These activities can be quite simple and routine as long as they are things that the fathers enjoy doing. The underlying theme for most of the coping strategies is to do something which is not part of the responsibilities related to work, taking care of household chores or supporting their wife and child. Professional life is deemed very helpful by some fathers as it allows them to take part in an activity that they like or that at least poses a different set of requirements on them compared to the role that they have to play at home. Sharing their experiences with others is also important in their ability to cope. It is important to note that as mentioned previously, it is not easy for the fathers to find others who they can talk to. However, whenever they get the opportunity to talk to someone who might be able to help—including friends, work colleagues, and even anonymous people on the internet—they share their experience with them, and it is always helpful.

Irrespective of the specific details of each situation and individual, the common element is an adoption of a positive outlook and holding on to hope with courage and resolve when they are facing some of the most challenging times of their lives. Aspects which could have been considered inconsequential previously now help the fathers when everything else around them seems to be disintegrating. For some fathers, it is a case of self-counselling, not losing hope and participating in any pleasurable activity no matter how small. However, coping involves a lot more than just the inward-facing strategies. It has an unmistakable element of social interaction and leaning upon sharing the experience with others in order to hear some words of encouragement to reinforce their courage and resolve.

Another important aspect is being vigilant about how to balance their needs and responsibilities. Fathers realise that it is impossible to meet all expectations and discharge all their responsibilities as a husband, father, breadwinner and homemaker at the same time. There are bound to be compromises along the way and occasionally the fathers have to disappoint someone to be able to cope with the demands of the situation. Being aware and finding the middle ground is very much part of the successful coping strategies. Existential philosophers—see, for example, Sartre (1946)—value the freedom to choose that individuals possess and their responsibility in the face of challenging circumstances. The fathers realize over time that they are free in their choices about how to respond to their difficulties and survive. The freedom of choice possessed by the individual is a fundamental existential concept; however, people may not be ready to accept the reality of this choice and may instead become depressed and desperate (Kierkegaard 1992; Nietzsche 2005). Or they might adhere to concepts that liberate them from their responsibility (Fromm 1941; Sartre 1946). The fathers realise that when they make their choices about what to prioritise, they face having to make compromises; however, acknowledging the reality and responsibility for these choices liberates them from feelings of depression and despair.

The essential elements that allow an individual to cope with the most difficult of circumstances are found to be commitment, control and challenge; and taken together, these are very close to Tillich's (1952) concept of the "courage to be". The fathers traverse the route of surviving in their situation by displaying the "courage to be" by leaning upon resilience through a combination of commitment, taking control and accepting the challenge. The attraction towards courage seems very important for the fathers. In a way, there is an equitability here with other great struggles that people face during their lives. We can find a homologue for the struggle of the fathers to cope with the challenges thrown their way, in the struggle of individuals who go to war. It conjures up images of men being tested, and of them discovering that they need other men to stand with them. As the experience matures and is assimilated, they also discover the importance of doing something so character forming, something which enhances the make-up of their self and results in personal growth. Existential philosophy is the philosophy of discord and strife, but also one of coping, boldness and managing (Kobasa 1982). For the fathers, coping with the challenge of circumstances facing them and finding ways of managing their own suffering as well as managing expectations and responsibilities on them from the social sphere of existence help them to grow as individuals and find new depths to their own self. Existential theorists have discussed a multitude of examples of individuals growing as a result of their sufferings and finding meaning from the suffering. If at the personal level an individual responds to suffering in the right way, with courage and resilience, then it possesses the potential to even bring benefits (Frankl 1962; Nietzsche 2005) and this certainly seems to be the case for fathers coping with the circumstances created when their partners suffered from PND.

Conclusion

The expansive scope of changes brought by the transition to parenthood can be challenging and whilst mothers are the primarily affected persons by PND, fathers are affected as well. Thus, PND affects the whole newly formed family (Halbreich 2005). The discussion above demonstrates the multidimensional, often challenging and prolonged struggle that fathers must face whilst their partners are suffering from PND. Their personal, social, physical and spiritual worlds undergo drastic changes. The fathers find themselves ill-equipped to deal with the situation because they are not aware of the impacts and implications of PND how it affects their partners deeply on an emotional level, making it hard to communicate openly and effectively. The relationship of both partners suffers greatly. Their emotional as well as physical well-being comes under immense pressure along with their partners, as the whole family tries to survive the difficult period and emerge successfully from the ordeal. Another factor that is important here are preconceived conceptions about the roles of fathers and mothers which need to be reconsidered in the newly changed family situation.

Understanding the experience of fathers living with partners suffering from PND can provide valuable information that can influence new proposals for healthcare provision and result in better-targeted support services and group work. Also, the particular sources of stress and anxiety, the feelings of loss, guilt, unfairness and other emotions highlighted by the findings of the current research can help to adapt therapeutic practices. There are unambiguous implications here about the need for better information and support provision to the parents-to-be, with healthcare staff playing an important role in that process. Also, it is clear that fathers lack a natural inclination towards asking for support, this coupled with a lack of readily available options contribute towards fathers suffering from a general lack of support during this difficult period. More awareness about the need to access support, and its benefits not only for the fathers, but also for the whole family, seems to be essential. At the same time, augmenting the knowledge base of health practitioners, counsellors and support providers is also a vital need because it can result in the provision of better-targeted care for the new fathers.

References

Buber, M. (1923/1958). *I and Thou* (2nd ed., R. G. Smith, Trans.). New York: Scribner.

Buber, M. (1970). *I and Thou* (W. Kaufmann, Trans., p. 57). New York: Charles Scribner's Sons.

Frankl, V. (1962). *Man's Search for Meaning*. New York: Touchstone Books.

Fromm, E. (1941). *Escape from Freedom*. New York: Rinehart & Co.

Halbreich, U. (2005). The Association Between Pregnancy Processes, Preterm Delivery, Low Birth Weight, and Postpartum Depressions—The Need for Interdisciplinary Integration. *American Journal of Obstetrics and Gynecology, 193*(4), 1312–1322.

Heidegger, M. (1927/1962). *Being and Time* (J. Macquarrie & E. Robinson, Trans.). San Francisco: Harper and Row.

Jaspers, K. (1941/1955). *Reason and Existenz* (W. Earle, Trans.). New York: Noonday Press.

Kierkegaard, S. (1992). *Eighteen Upbuilding Discourses* (No. 5). Princeton: Princeton University Press.

Kobasa, S. C. (1982). Commitment and Coping in Stress Resistance Among Lawyers. *Journal of Personality and Social Psychology, 42*(4), 707.

Nietzsche, F. (2005). *Thus Spoke Zarathustra* (G. Parkes, Trans.). Oxford: Oxford University Press.

Prinds, C., Hvidt, N. C., Mogensen, O., & Buus, N. (2013). Making Existential Meaning in Transition to Motherhood: A Scoping Review. *Midwifery*. https://doi.org/10.1016/j.midw.2013.06.021.

Robertson, E., Grace, S., Wallington, T., & Stewart, D. E. (2004). Antenatal Risk Factors for Postpartum Depression: A Synthesis of Recent Literature. *General Hospital Psychiatry, 26*(4), 289–295.

Sadia, F. (2020). *A Phenomenological Exploration into the Lived Experience of Fathers Living with New Mothers Diagnosed as PND* (Doctoral dissertation). Middlesex University and New School of Psychotherapy and Counselling.

Sartre, J. (1939). *Sketch for a Theory of the Emotions* (P. Mairet, Trans.). London: Methuen.

Sartre, J. P. (1946/1948). *Existentialism and Humanism* (P. Mairet, Trans.). London: Methuen.

Tillich, P. (1952). *The Courage to Be*. New Haven, CT: Yale University Press.

Van Deurzen, E. (1997). *Everyday Mysteries: Existential Dimensions of Psychotherapy*. London: Routledge.

Van Deurzen, E. (2012). *Existential Counselling & Psychotherapy in Practice*. London: Sage.

Van Deurzen-Smith, E. (1988). *Existential Counselling in Practice*. London: Sage.

Wong, P. T., Wong, L. C., & Scott, C. (2006). Beyond Stress and Coping: The Positive Psychology of Transformation. In *Handbook of Multicultural Perspectives on Stress and Coping* (pp. 1–26). Boston, MA: Springer.

Part III

Social Crisis: An Existential Understanding of the Impact on Motherhood of Social and Cultural Aspects

10

Identity and Mothering: The Second Generation of Ghanaian Migrants

Jennifer Ofori

Introduction

Within the vast literature that exists on the experiences of motherhood, there has been little written about the experiences of motherhood for ethnic minority women living in the United Kingdom (henceforth UK) (Lim 2012). Roy Moodley (2006) argues that research amongst the black and ethnic minority group in the counselling profession is 'marginal, underfunded and not taken seriously by the counselling and psychotherapy research community' (Moodley cited in Lago 2006: 229–271). Topics involving 'culture and the family functioning' of black and ethnic minority populations are rarely ever explored from a qualitative research perspective (ibid.: 237). Of the research which remains currently available, many of the studies appear to have focused on measuring the parenting styles of ethnic minority families from a quantitative research perspective (Phoenix and Husain 2007) or have researched numerous ethnic minority mothers rather than looking at individual groups within

J. Ofori (✉)
London, UK

C. Arnold-Baker (ed.), *The Existential Crisis of Motherhood*,
https://doi.org/10.1007/978-3-030-56499-5_10

this diverse population (Hollway 2015). However, more research is needed to understand the uniquely diverse cultural experiences of ethnic minority parents in the UK, from a culturally specific perspective.

Due to an absence of literature surrounding this particular group of British mothers, it was clear a study which explored the identities and mothering practices of a black British ethnic minority group of mothers from an existential phenomenological perspective was needed to address this gap. This chapter is therefore focused on offering an existential understanding of the mothering experiences of an ethnic minority group of British mothers who are of second-generation Ghanaian descent. The chapter will review the meaning of first-time motherhood from various disciplines, before focussing on relevant research regarding the motherhood experiences of mothers from black ethnic minority backgrounds resident in the UK. This will form the background to the phenomenological research presented in this chapter. The chapter will conclude with a discussion on the implications for practice.

'Identity' in First-Time Mothers

Biological Perspective

The process of becoming a mother has first and foremost always been viewed and acknowledged as a biological given, due to the role that biology plays in the woman's ability to reproduce (Romito 1997). It is evident that there is indeed a biological and medical facet to becoming a mother as stated by psychologist Romito, who stressed an entanglement between the identity of women and their roles in the reproductive process. However, not all women opt to become mothers and the ones that do may encounter differing experiences.

> Mothers are often confronted with an array of public and lay knowledge through which their expectations and experiences of motherhood will have been mediated prior to and throughout the process of reproduction. (Miller 2000: 1)

The biological perspective has, therefore, been helpful in identifying general experiences and describing the process of becoming a mother from a medical viewpoint but offers very little in the area of 'identity' for first-time mothers.

Sociological and Anthropological Perspectives

A plethora of sociological and anthropological approaches have sought to explore the impact that societal and cultural differences may have on mothering identities and the choices that are implemented by first-time mothers, living in a variety of cultures (Romito 1997; Miller 2000; Doswell 2001; Stopford 2007; Mantovani 2010; Quinn and Mageo 2013). Of the research in existence, there has been an acknowledgement of the differences existing between the choices of mothering styles and the practices of women living in various African countries (Quinn and Mageo 2013) compared to mothers from Western societies. These studies have shown that the practice of mothering and the meanings derived from the mothering journey are socially and culturally specific.

Psychological Perspective

Researchers within the psychological field (Klein 1932; Winnicott 1971; Stern 1995; Priel and Besser 2001; Mayo and Moutsou 2017) have also offered varied perspectives on the topic of motherhood to gain an understanding of the emotional and psychological facets of the experience of motherhood for first-time mothers. One such researcher, the psychoanalyst Daniel Stern, proposed that following the birth of a baby, the mother passes into a psychic organisation called the 'motherhood constellation' (Stern 1995: 171). He describes this constellation as a 'psychic organiser' (ibid.), which leads to the realignment of the new mother's sense of individual identity, as a separate entity to that of her mothering role. He describes this process as one whereby an internal and external process of psychic discourse is attempted between the new mother and herself, the new mother and her baby, and between the new mother and her own mother, in relation to how she was mothered as a child.

Stern's contributions have successfully highlighted the psychological and identity challenges faced by first-time mothers as they adapt to their new role. The identities that first-time mothers will go on to possess will largely be influenced by how each mother processes her emotional and psychological feelings on becoming a mother.

Existential Perspective

Very little has been written about the topic of motherhood from an existential perspective, of the sparse literature in existence it has been noted that becoming a mother is a life-altering subjective experience. It is subjective in that each mother is individual, and as experiences may differ from one mother to the next, they therefore cannot be objectively defined. Butterfield suggests that motherhood is ambiguous in that it is both determined, due to 'the physical realities of the mothering process' and 'individually freeing' (Butterfield 2010: 67–68), as the mothering experience remains open to societal, cultural, historical and individual influences.

Prinds et al. (2013) conducted a scoping review of pre-existing research related to the transition to motherhood in the West. Eleven studies, conducted between 1990 and 2010, from Europe, Russia, North America and Australia were selected in order to explore how mothers of full-term babies made existential meaning in their 'transitions to motherhood in western oriented countries' (Prinds et al. 2013: 735). van Deurzen's (2005) four dimensions of existence was utilised in their analysis (van Deurzen and Arnold-Baker 2005). Overall, their scoping review concluded that motherhood is an existentially challenging experience, which causes mothers to re-evaluate and redefine the meanings of their new worlds, following the birth of their babies. Motherhood, therefore, represents a life transition, which leads to the mother's overall assessment of her identity, values and meanings.

More recently, Arnold-Baker (2015) explored the existential dimensions of the transition to motherhood of eight first-time mothers whose babies were aged between 6 and 12 months. Her study found that each of the mothers reported changes to life as they knew it and changes to their experiences of themselves. It also revealed that on becoming mothers for the first time, the mothers highlighted the importance of seeking social forms of support. The mothers described having to redefine their social relationships, their sense of their values, beliefs, expectations and self-identities, and they became confronted with previously unaware aspects of 'freedom, choice and responsibility' (Arnold-Baker 2015: 2) within their mothering roles.

The existential perspective acknowledges that the transition to motherhood is a life transition that should be recognised as a complex phenomenon, which challenges each dimension of any mother's existence. Motherhood is subjective, as the experiences faced by each mother will be different. The meanings derived from the experience will be dependent on how the mother processes her transition, chooses to identify or position herself in her role and how she faces the challenges to previously upheld values, beliefs and/or expectations.

What Is Known About Black Ethnic Minority Mothers in the UK?

As previously stated, there remains a significant gap in the literature regarding mothers belonging to the British ethnic minority population group, currently resident in the UK. Of the studies in existence, I have chosen to reflect on two studies, which offer insight into the cultural experiences of black ethnic minority mothers from a UK perspective.

The first of these studies, by Reynolds (1998), aimed to construct a discourse on what it meant to be a black mother in the UK. She interviewed twenty African-Caribbean mothers using a semi-structured free flowing interviewing style. Despite the various differences amongst the mothers, such as: their ages, marital status, social class and generational differences, which may have heavily influenced their mothering experiences, she found four mothering identity factors, which united their experiences collectively. These were

1. the way in which their 'mothering was informed by a re-constituted collective Caribbean identity, which relied on memory and re-memory in order to re-construct itself' (Reynolds 1998: 325);
2. the ways in which these mothers individually engaged 'in creating diverse childrearing strategies to challenge and resist racism' (ibid.);
3. the role that a work identity had in influencing their overall African-Caribbean mothering identities and lastly;
4. the impact that black African-Caribbean fathering had on their identities, mothering experiences and their social constructions of their mothering identities (ibid.).

As part of her conclusion, Reynolds reflected that in order to understand the true nature of mothering experiences, 'homogeneous and stereotypical images of black and white mothering, should be separated' (ibid.). She advocated the use of a universal mothering model, which allowed for an exploration of 'the mothering experiences of all women to be heard' (ibid.: 335); however, this is a model that has yet to be executed. Despite a lack of a focused participant selection criteria, a limitation of Reynolds' study (as mothers belonged to the first, second or third generation of British Caribbean population group were permitted to participate in the study, irrespective of their diverse generational group identities), her overall contribution has been particularly useful in highlighting how important it is for the lived experiences of all mothers to be explored.

In 2010, Mantovani set out to explore 'the experiences of fifteen young black single, teenage mothers who were being looked after by their local authority' (Mantovani 2010: 3). She found that the mothers all seemed to experience stigma, shame and blame, but responded to this in differing ways. Whilst a proportion of the mothers in her study rejected their perceived 'public identity', to validate their own sense of identity, some mothers appeared to embrace a 'self-limiting identity' (ibid.: 237, 249). They all experienced 'identity conflicts' where their 'sense of self-identity clashed with their perceived social identities' (ibid.) which were projected on to them by others in their external environments.

The findings from both Reynolds' and Montavani's studies highlight the impact that societal expectations can have on a mothers' identity and choice of mothering practices. Both studies shed light on the individual experiences of a population of black and/or African-Caribbean mothers. However, their lack of homogeneity in the selection of their participants will most certainly have influenced their personal journeys into motherhood dramatically and therefore their overall findings. Nonetheless, these studies have demonstrated a need to explore the individual mothering experiences of ethnic minority mothers of first, second or even third generations further.

Identity and Mothering: The Second Generation of Ghanaian Migrants

The current study, from which this chapter is centred, was therefore undertaken with the aim of exploring, clarifying and describing the phenomenon of 'self-identity' and its influence on the mothering practices of an ethnic minority group of mothers from an existential phenomenological perspective.

Background to the Study

March the 30th 2011, the date on which my daughter was born, signified the start of a philosophical journey of what it meant to become a mother for the first time. In giving birth to my daughter I unwittingly gave birth to my identity of mother, a deeply profound experience that could not have been fully anticipated nor premeditated.

I had started to feel pressured by my mother's cultural expectations of the appropriate ways to care for my child, which appeared to be different from the information and advice that had been provided by the health care professionals I came into contact with. In feeling disconnected from my mother, I started questioning my relationship to her and my Ghanaian culture. During this time, I became struck by a newspaper report in the *Guardian* Newspaper (2011) detailing the case of a baby whose mother; 'a 31 year old nurse of Ghanaian descent who had been residing in the United Kingdom for approximately 9 years' (Waltham

Forest Safeguarding Children Board Executive Summary 2011: 2) had been found guilty of force-feeding her child to death (Davies 2011). What caused this case to stand out for me was her insistence that her force-feeding practice had been reflective of her cultural upbringing and not an intentional act to hurt her child.

This case led me to reflect on my own mothering experience, as a second-generation Ghanaian migrant because it demonstrated the impact that 'perceived' cultural norms, expectations and values, can have on the way a mother may choose to care for her child. It raised a number of questions which led to the inspiration to embark on a heuristic exploration of my own mothering experience alongside the accounts of eight other British mothers of second-generation Ghanaian descent. The mothers were between the ages of 23 and 42 at the time of their interviews and had become mothers at different ages (with two becoming first-time mothers aged 16 and 17, a limitation of the study). They identified as first-time mothers with children between the ages of 2 and 10. Irrespective of these distinctions, there were no overall differences in the themes identified between any of the participants interviewed. Three themes were identified: '*Identity: The self as creation*', '*Mothering Practices: Finding meaning in mothering*' and '*Influence: Being in relation to others*' and they describe the mothering experiences of these nine first-time mothers (myself included).

Identity

Early Childhood Perceptions

The findings demonstrated that identity is a complex phenomenon, which is subject to adaptation or individual preference. The majority of the mothers interviewed in the study found their merged British-Ghanaian identity difficult to grasp during the earlier stages of their childhood. Rather than viewing their British identities and Ghanaian cultural influences in a combined way, the mothers admitted to viewing their identities in singular form (as either solely Ghanaian or solely British) as a way of responding to their ethnic and cultural differences from the majority of the British population. With some believing that the colour of their skin and/or their cultural differences identified them as being different from their peers and from the rest of the British population. This was reflected by some of the mothers' narratives:

> ***Adwoa-*** *'...growing up I felt like I was British especially as I lived in this country'.* (Ofori 2018: 105)
> ***Yaa Adoma-*** *'I mean as a child I wanted to blend in with the rest'.* (ibid.)
> ***Akosua-*** *'...when I was younger because I was so young and my parents were from Ghana I just used to feel Ghanaian through and through, because it was just easier to think I was from Ghana'.* (ibid.: 106)
> ***Jennifer-*** *'I never considered myself British. I didn't think I could be British because of the colour of my skin, I felt that I was from Ghana and that I was Ghanaian because of my family's heritage and culture'.* (ibid.)

The 'Self' as a Creation

When viewing identity from an existential lens, 'self as a creation' represented the way in which the mothers were able to describe how their perceptions of 'self' evolved over time. The phenomenon of 'Identity' for most of the mothers had been perceived to be one which needed to be 'objectively defined' (Sartre 2010) in an either-or dichotomy initially. The mothers admitted to wanting to categorise themselves during the earlier stages of their lives.

Of those mothers who struggled to grasp their British-Ghanaian identity in equal measure during the earlier stages of childhood, a shift appears to have occurred at some point prior to motherhood. Whereby rather than viewing their identities as '*singular*', the mothers began to view them from a '*merged*' British-Ghanaian cultural perspective. It was interesting to note that despite the mothers' initial conceptions of their identities, they all described their present identities as equally representing their British and Ghanaian influences, having appeared to have merged both identities together. This is demonstrated below by three of the mothers:

> ***Ama***- *'…we are British but we are Ghanaians in Britain and you know regardless of the fact that I wasn't born there it is a part of me…it's the only thing that I can identify with'.* (Ofori 2018: 108)
> **Adwoa**- *'Right now I consider myself to be both and I genuinely believe that yes I am both…. I… am… tweaking bits that I like'.* (ibid.)
> ***Akosua***- *'I can't say I am just British or just Ghanaian, I am basically in the middle and I have found my own way of being both'.* (ibid.: 109)

The mothers reflected on how their merged British-Ghanaian identities had evolved over time and their perceptions of their identities had changed from their adolescent years. The mothers viewed their identities from a purely individual perspective, although most found it difficult to articulate what their merged British-Ghanaian identities meant to them. As shown in the following extracts:

> ***Ama***- *'…we are British but we are Ghanaians in Britain and you know regardless of the fact that I wasn't born there it is a part of me…it's the only thing that I can identify with'.* (ibid.: 108)
> **Adwoa**- *'Right now I consider myself to be both and I genuinely believe that yes I am both…. I… am… tweaking bits that I like'.* (ibid.)
> ***Akosua***- *'I can't say I am just British or just Ghanaian, I am basically in the middle and I have found my own way of being both'.* (ibid.: 109)

These findings coincide with Sartre's views of 'self' which suggests that the human being is 'thrown into a world…abandoned in a situation' (Sartre 2010: 103), exists in the world and is responsible for creating an essence or an identity 'for-itself' (ibid.). This was particularly the case for the mothers of this study, as they seemed to be actively creating a newly distinct merged mothering identity, by fusing their British-Ghanaian influences together. This can also be viewed from the perspective of the *Eigenwelt* or personal world, which represents the dimension of the 'private self' of the individual and our 'existence with ourselves' (van Deurzen and Arnold-Baker 2005: 157). Our sense of self is created out of our experiences and interactions and involves a process of self-reflection. Therefore, each mother's identities are personal to themselves and not purely representative of their racial–cultural group memberships or associations. The mothers had responded to their social identities in a creative way, by incorporating their merged identities into their mothering roles.

Mothering Practices

The findings highlighted the importance of support, for each of the mothers interviewed during the initial phases of their babies' lives. The mothers admitted to drawing on the support of their own mothers, aunts and/or health care practitioners for encouragement, following the birth of their babies. In some cultures, mothers are given extra support to help them adjust to their mothering roles (Kruchman 1992), and this was particularly the case for the mothers in this current study. They opted to participate in the child rearing practices and/or ceremonies specific to their Ghanaian culture, as demonstrated by their own mothers (who were first-generation Ghanaian migrants living in the UK).

Previous literature and research on first-time mothers (Kruchman 1992; Stern 1995; Miller 2000; Arnold-Baker 2015; Hollway 2015) have also highlighted the importance of mothers' need for support from others, during the initial stages of their mothering journeys. Although the practices enacted by most of the mothers interviewed seemed to represent a Ghanaian child rearing preference, each of the mothers felt the need to gain extra forms of support as they were unsure about their mothering practices and were attempting to identify their own mothering preferences. This support was either from their mothers, health care professionals or drawing on previous experiences, i.e. from knowledge of seeing other mothers caring for their babies, for the most appropriate child rearing care practices.

Birth of 'Mother'

The majority of the mothers in this study sought the support of their own mothers, who they felt were more experienced and could therefore help them to enact the basic new-born Ghanaian nurturing methods they felt were required, although, with a cultural twist. The mothers were caught in an ambiguous tension (Butterfield 2010), where they felt bound by culturally distinct basic methods which were required in the nurturing of a new-born baby and which held significance for their Ghanaian heritage; yet they also felt there was flexibility in how these methods could be employed. This tension highlighted the ambiguous nature of motherhood for these mothers, how they felt determined by their heritage and yet free to choose how they lived that heritage. Four mothers explained this further:

> ***Efya-*** *'Initially I did have a huge amount of support from my mum, she was sort of teaching me on the job… I mean my mum was pretty adamant… she taught me how to clean the belly button area, she taught me how to bath the baby with Shea butter…'* (Ofori 2018: 110)
> **Ama-** *'…my son was predominantly breastfed initially,… and I brought him up more traditionally as a Ghanaian. So things like when he was born… arranging his circumcision, massaging his legs, stretching his limbs and his body, shaping his head… my mum…is a born and bred Ghanaian so she would do or encourage me to do things her way'.* (ibid.: 81)
> **Adwoa-** *'I used to explain it to people at work they would say some weird things you know as they would imagine that my mother would…take over every aspect of taking care of my child…it is more of a partnership…so what you do is you shape the head and you kind of like stretch the limbs and you massage the body and…he was even circumcised'.* (ibid.: 111)
> ***Abena-*** *'Well because I was young and my mum had passed away, the health care professionals visited us twice a week but when I would explain how I bath the baby they would say: you shouldn't stretch the limbs you will cause the baby harm!'.* (ibid.: 98)

The mothers initially appeared to proceed on their mothering journey trusting in the 'objectively' defined illusion of the mothering process (De Beauvoir 1956) as proposed by those around them. But were then confronted with the reality of its flexibility, due to the differences in the cultural practices being implemented by significant family members. This finding confirms previous existential research (Arnold-Baker 2015; Prinds et al. 2013), which suggested the importance of social support for first-time mothers during the initial stages of their mothering journey.

It also links to Deurzen's concept of the *Mitwelt* or the social dimension, which represents our 'existence with others' (van Deurzen 2002: 135). Mothers connect with their own mothers and other public forms of support (health care practitioners), and these connections have an impact on how the woman enacts her mothering during their initial transitions.

By interacting in differing social modes, the mothers engage in a comparing and contrasting process during which they choose to alter their way of mothering to discover their personal preferences. This finding therefore stresses the importance of health care workers and practitioners of all capacities, in providing a supportive environment for new mothers.

Family Preservation Through Food

'Family preservation through food' refers to the ways in which the mothers were attempting to preserve their cultural and familial identities by upholding culinary delicacies in the context of their wider family group settings.

When discussing their current mothering practices of 'food preparations', most of the mothers admitted that they are not currently cooking solely Ghanaian dishes but instead were either merging their two cultures together or cooking solely British dishes. Yet each of them stressed that they enjoyed indulging in Ghanaian culinary preferences when in the company of their Ghanaian mothers and wider family groups, therefore acknowledging both aspects of their identities, as opposed to placing one identity above the other. By indulging in the culinary dishes of their Ghanaian culture in the presence of family members, they had found a way of keeping their Ghanaian identities alive in the present. This was demonstrated in the following transcripts:

> ***Akua-*** *'I find that I am cooking more British or western dishes... when we are at home we are eating more British or western food, like shepherds pie, a pizza, and roast or what ever else. But I'm finding that when I'm with my mum weekly...I love Ghanaian food and I much rather like to eat Ghanaian food'.* (Ofori 2018: 113)

> ***Esi-*** *'She eats more British foods like spaghetti and mash potato when she's with me but when we go to my mums, my mum will give her Kenkey or Chicken'.* (ibid.: 114)
> ***Adowa-*** *'I'm not sure if this is specifically Ghanaian but in my household we definitely have more of a spicier pallet and so my son had to embrace that… he knows how to eat with his hand and he likes Jollof too… I would say here take a little bit… until eventually he started to prefer spice… He has got to be able to eat our food because if he goes to an aunt's house he needs to be able to eat what is being cooked'.* (ibid.)

Food performed an important function for these mothers, as it brought together the physical, social and personal dimensions of their existence. Food not only nourishes and provides sustenance for the family, but it can be a social event whereby family members and friends are brought together, and it is also a way in which the mothers were able to express a sense of their identity. 'Food', therefore, became an 'objective' anchor for this group of mothers, which helped to consolidate their merged identities in a physical form.

This finding highlights the importance of the *Umwelt* or physical dimension of existence for these mothers and offers practitioners working with ethnic minorities, a new and distinct avenue of exploration.

Cultural Tensions: Education and Discipline

Each mother embarked on a process of reflection of their own experiences of being parented as well as how they were also exercising their personal parenting preferences.

When discussing their attitudes towards education, each of the mothers admitted to viewing education as an important and essential factor in determining their child's future success. A view which they suggest had been influenced by their Ghanaian cultural upbringing and one based on how they were parented by their Ghanaian parents. An example of this is expressed below:

Akua- *'My mum was very Ghanaian... I mean she was very strict, very disciplined, very focused on education...I'm taking my cue from my experiences and the way that my mother has raised me'.* (ibid.: 115)

Adwoa- *'I think education is something that should be appreciated and I share that message to my son, he needs to appreciate the opportunities available...it is not always about being academic...he can be an athlete, or a designer or a creator. I am going to let my son be creative...it is a merge of my personal experience'.* (ibid.: 116)

Similarly, when discussing parental attitudes towards discipline, each of the mothers stressed the importance of 'discipline' for their children. 'Discipline' was viewed by each as a vital child rearing practice, which acted as a boundary reinforcement tool and helped to instil values of respect. This was a view that all admitted had been influenced by their parents' and Ghanaian culture in general.

This illuminated the importance of education and discipline for members of the British-Ghanaian second generation. The mothers appeared to be engaging in a 'psychic discourse' (Stern 2010) with themselves whereby they re-engaged with their childhood experiences and reflected over their own mother's attitudes towards both these areas. This was the backdrop against which they decoded which mothering practices to continue or which to adapt. This is expressed below:

Ama- *'I am not going to be critical of how other people deal with their child or children but for my son and I we have to be able to sit on the table and I have to be able to show you how, or where you've gone wrong. I get angry just like everybody else, but I think some of the lengths that I've seen used in the past from specific Ghanaians are extreme'.* (Ofori 2018: 118)

Abena- *'Discipline is a must and I am a believer in being firm. Not in the same way that it was like when I was a child with being physically beaten, but that in my child knowing my look and not talking back. For me respecting your elders is an important boundary...it is definitely my Ghanaian influence...I don't feel a need to put my hand on my child for her to be respectful, communication is enough'.* (ibid.: 119)

Efya- *'It's a lot stricter in Ghanaian or even an African household...I take fundamental elements from my own family's choice of upbringing and small elements from the British influence.* (ibid.: 118)

The process of reflection that took place for these first-time mothers demonstrated that they were constantly having to engage with these tensions in the *Eigenwelt* or personal and the *Uberwelt* or spiritual dimensions (van Deurzen 2002). In order to re-evaluate and redefine the meanings of their mothering journey's, this re-evaluation enabled the mothers to represent their two cultures and incorporate them in an individually freeing and meaningful way.

Finding Meaning in Mothering: Adaptation and Continuation

The mothers went through a process of reflection, adaptation and continuation as they reflected on being parented themselves. They had to choose whether to continue to hold on to their parents' way of parenting or adapt their mothering. This was not an either/or choice but came out of reflection, personal preferences, and by making active choices which meant the mothers found a personally meaningful way to be a mother.

Rather than viewing their present-day mothering practices as 'fixed' and determined, as had previously been anticipated during the early phases of their transition, the first-time mothers began exercising their personal freedoms. They were choosing to mother in ways that they found personally meaningful, in spite of their past experiences and cultural influences. Some of the mothers admitted to feeling inspired by the approaches enacted by their own parents and therefore choose to repeat those same parental styles and attitudes, particularly towards education and discipline, whereas a proportion of the mothers interviewed appeared to be implementing adjustments to their parent's attitudes, based on their own personal preferences and experiences.

This finding is particularly distinct as it showed that regardless of how long women had been mothers (a combined maximum period of up to ten years as their children were between the ages of 2 and 10 at the time of the interview,) they continued to be actively immersed in their mothering roles and immersed in this process of reflection. This also reinforced an existential perspective that individuals have the potential to continually engage with their personal 'freedoms', 'responsibilities', and 'choices' and in doing so create 'meaning' for themselves (Sartre 2010).

Influence

It was revealed that when discussing their present-day mothering influences, the majority of the mothers (excluding two) stated that their partners, siblings and/or other family members, religious groups, wider community groups and/or colleagues from work influenced aspects of their mothering choices and decisions.

Being in Relation to 'Others'

'Being in relation to others' refers to the social dimension of mothering, where each mother seemed to draw on their social relationships for support with their mothering queries or concerns. It was through these relationships that they found a way to make their experiences more meaningful.

Existential philosophy acknowledges that we are social beings immersed in the world with 'others' (Heidegger 1962; Sartre 2010; van Deurzen 2002). The dimension of the *Mitwelt* suggests that we exist in a 'with-world' (van Deurzen and Arnold-Baker 2005: 89) amongst others where we attempt to compare and contrast ourselves by responding to the social, cultural and political environments in which we are 'embedded' (van Deurzen 2002: 69). The mothers exist in a social–cultural context from which they have chosen their own mothering practices.

For this group of mothers then, the *Mitwelt* or social dimension appears to be an important factor that contributes to the mothering styles that are adopted. Although this was not the case for all mothers (i.e. two out of the nine mothers interviewed), it was certainly the case for the others, both in the initial stages of their mothering journeys and beyond.

Each of the mothers responded to their British-Ghanaian culturally influenced mothering identity, in ways that they found personally meaningful. This aspect was represented in the *Uberwelt* dimension or the spiritual world. Deurzen's (2005) *Uberwelt* represents the dimension of the ideological beliefs and values of a person's 'life, the world, themselves and beyond' and happens to symbolise 'the domain of experience where people create meaning for themselves and make sense of things' (van Deurzen, 2002: 86–87).

Therefore, this finding revealed that first-time mothers of second-generation Ghanaian descent are engaging in the '*Mitwelt*' when making their mothering decisions, but they are not bound to the suggestions or influences of their family members or wider community. Rather, these mothers admit that they are also engaging in the '*Uberwelt*' dimension when assessing their core beliefs and adapting their mothering practices to reflect them. Mothering for this group of women is experienced as a freedom inducing experience, which is subject to individual modification.

Conclusion

With growing numbers of mothers of mixed cultural backgrounds living in the UK, there is a need for practitioners working with this client group to think more closely about the psycho-social–cultural and existential dimensions of their clients' worlds. This study also emphasises the importance of exploring the intergenerational facets of their clients' heritage when working with ethnic minority members.

The study revealed that identity is a complex phenomenon, which can only be understood at an individual level, where cultural background meets everyday living. The accounts of the nine British mothers (researcher included) in this study indicated that mothers who are second-generation British-Ghanaian identify equally as British and Ghanaian. These mothers described their merged British-Ghanaian identities and disclosed how their merged identities had evolved over time.

From an existential perspective, the current study reiterated and added to the findings of previous studies, which emphasised that motherhood is an existentially altering experience, which sparks continuous changes on all dimensions of each mother's existence. However, this was also shown to be true for the mothers' identity, each dimension represented a different aspect of the mothers' emerging identity. The Umwelt or physical dimension was represented through food preparation and feeding the family. The women disclosed that on becoming mothers, their merged British-Ghanaian identities were reflected in their cooking preferences. 'Food' was viewed by this group of mothers as an 'objective' anchor, which helped to keep their merged identities alive, in a physical form—an outward portrayal of their internal representations.

There was also a social dimension to this mothering journey, which began from the moment the child was born. This study revealed that in the dimension of the *Mitwelt* (social dimension), the mothers underwent a process of self-reflection which they engaged in continuously over time. Rather than remaining defined by their racial, intergenerational or cultural group associations and/or memberships, the mothers were able to respond to their identities creatively. Their social context becoming the background onto which they created themselves anew. This aspect of the mothers' identity was also part of the *Eigenwelt* (personal dimension), where the mothers were able to take responsibility for the sense of themselves that they were creating.

The *Uberwelt* (spiritual dimension) was represented through the mothers' values and beliefs and how they created meaning for themselves and their experiences. The mothers assessed their core beliefs and adapted their mothering practices to reflect them. Mothering for this group was experienced as a freedom inducing experience, which was subject to individual modification as each mother responded to their British-Ghanaian culturally influenced mothering identities, in ways that they found personally meaningful.

The mothering journey for these mothers was therefore one, which remained in continuous flux and subject to change, as their journeys unfolded, and their children developed. Practitioners should keep this in mind when working with British ethnic groups. To gain a deeper understanding of their experience, a four-dimension model is suggested, to highlight the ways in which mothers merge their cultural heritage with their current context to form a meaningful sense of themselves as mothers. There is a need for support groups for ethnic minority mothers which would offer these mothers the opportunity to reflect on their mothering experiences in a non-judgemental setting. As this study has shown, these groups would also be needed for those further into their motherhood journeys beyond the initial postnatal phase.

References

Arnold-Baker, C. (2015). *How Becoming a Mother Involves a Confrontation with Existence: An Existential Phenomenological Exploration of the Experience of Early Motherhood* [Online]. Available from: http://eprints.mdx.ac.uk/18278/1/CArnoldBakerThesis.pdf. Accessed February 6, 2016.

Butterfield, E. (2010). Days and Nights of a New Mother: Existentialism in the Nursery. In S. Lintott (Ed.), *Motherhood: Philosophy for Everyone*. West Sussex: Wiley.

Davies, C. (2011). Mother Found Guilty of Force-Feeding Baby to Death. *The Guardian* [Online]. Available from: http://www.theguardian.com/uk/2011/oct/12/mother-force-feeding-baby-death?view=mobile. Accessed March 1, 2013.

De Beauvoir, S. (1956). *The Second Sex*. London: Lowe and Brydone Ltd.

Doswell, B. (2001). *Born In Britain: The Lost Generation—A Study of Young Black People in Croydon, the Children of Immigrants from the Caribbean.* London: Brunel University.

Heidegger, M. (1962). *Being in Time*. Oxford: Basil Blackwall Publisher Ltd.

Hollway, W. (2015). *Knowing Mothers: Researching Maternal Identity Change*. Hampshire: Palgrave Macmillan.

Klein, M. (1932). *The Psycho-Analysis of Children*. London: Hogarth Press and the Institute of Psycho-Analysis.

Kruchman, L. D. (1992). Rituals and Support: An Anthropological View of Postpartum Depression. In J. Hamilton & P. Harberger (Eds.), *Postpartum Psychiatric Illness: A Picture Puzzle*. USA: University of Pennsylvania Press.

Lago, R. (2006). Race, Culture and Counselling Challenge In: The Ongoing Challenge. In R. Moodley & V. Clemmont (Eds.), *Race and Culture in Counselling Research*. Buckingham: Open University Press.

Lim, H. (2012). *The Intersection of Motherhood Identity with Culture and Class: A Qualitative Study of East Asian Mothers in England*. Bath, UK: University of Bath.

Mayo, R., & Moutsou, C. (2017). *The Mother In Psychoanalysis and Beyond: Matricide and Maternal Subjectivity*. London: Routledge.

Miller, A. T. (2000). *An Exploration of First Time Motherhood: Narratives of Transition*. Warwick, UK: University of Warwick.

Montavani, N. (2010). *Identity Work, Moral Accountability and Good Mothering Practices in Narratives of Black Teenaged Mothers*. London: Royal Holloway University.

Ofori, J. (2018). *Identity and Mothering: The Second Generation of Ghanaian Migrants*. London: Middlesex University.

Phoenix, A., & Husain, Y. (2007). *Parenting and Ethnicity*. York: Joseph Rowntree Foundation.

Phoenix, A., Woollett, A., & Lloyd, E. (1991). *Motherhood: Meanings, Practices and Ideologies*. London: Sage.

Priel, B., & Besser, A. (2001). Bridging the Gap Between Attachment and Object Relations Theories: A Study of the Transition to Motherhood. *British Journal of Medical Psychology, 74*(2001), 85–100.

Prinds, C., Hvidt, N. C., Mogensen, O., & Buus, N. (2013). Making Existential Meaning in Transition to Motherhood: A Scoping Review. *Midwifery* [Online]. Available from: http://dx.doi.org/10.1016/j.midw.2013.06.021. Accessed October 27, 2015.

Quinn, N., & Mageo, J. (Eds.). (2013). *Attachment Reconsidered: Cultural Perspectives on a Western Theory*. Hampshire: Palgrave.

Reynolds, A. T. (1998). *African-Caribbean Mothering: Re-Constructing a 'New' Identity*. London: Southbank University.

Romito, P. (1997). Damned If You Do and Damned If You Don't: Psychological and Social Constraints on Motherhood in Contemporary Europe. In A. Oakley & J. Mitchell (Eds.), *Who's Afraid of Feminism? Seeing Through the Backlash*. London: Hamish Hamilton.

Sartre, J. P. (2003). *Being and Nothingness*. Abingdon: Routledge.

Sartre, P. J. (2010). *Being and Nothingness*. Abingdon: Routledge.

Stern, N. D. (1995). *The Motherhood Constellation: A Unified View of Psychotherapy*. London: Karnac.

Stopford, A. (2007). *Mothering Children of African Descent: Hopes, fears and strategies of White Birth Mothers*. Sydney: University of Western Sydney.

van Deurzen, E. (2002). *Existential Counselling and Psychotherapy in Practice*. London: Sage.

van Deurzen, E., & Adams, M. (2011). *Skills in Existential Counselling and Psychotherapy*. London: Sage.
van Deurzen, E., & Arnold-Baker, C. (2005). *Existential Perspectives on Human Issues: A Handbook for Therapeutic Practice*. Hampshire: Palgrave Macmillan.
Waltham Forest Safeguarding Children Board Executive Summary. (2011). *Serious Case Review*. Available from: http://www.walthamforest.gov.uk/Documents/2011_10_21_executive_summary_child_w_v4_-_final.pdf.
Winnicott, W. D. (1971). *Playing and Reality*. London: Routledge.

11

Motherhood and the Traumatic Death of One's Child

Susan Harris

Introduction

> Your child is not something you can kind of let go of whether they're alive or dead they're kind of always with you and just because he's dead doesn't mean that he's not with me. (Sophie)

Traumatic bereavement refers to a sudden, unexpected death, often in violent or frightening circumstances, this may include fatal accidents: drowning, car accident, violent deaths by murder, suicide, and natural sudden deaths, or preventable deaths for example, from medical error (Rando 1993; Rynearson et al. 2013). Bereavement is considered one of the most painful and distressing of all human experiences (Bowlby 1980). However, a traumatic bereavement brings its own unique set of challenges. The death of a child in developed countries is viewed as tragic and against the natural order of life, in contrast to developing countries

S. Harris (✉)
London, UK

C. Arnold-Baker (ed.), *The Existential Crisis of Motherhood*,
https://doi.org/10.1007/978-3-030-56499-5_11

where child mortality rates are high, and the death of a child is experienced as a more common part of life, which influences sociocultural beliefs and attitudes towards child loss and parental mourning (Gorer 1987; Young and Papadatou 1997). Western research has identified that the death of a child creates an 'empty space' for bereaved family members (McClowry et al. 1987). The bereaved parent's life is forever changed, and life will never be the same again (Seigal 2017). There is no question that the death of a child is experienced as the most profoundly painful, and devastating life-altering experience for a parent, however, when the death is experienced in traumatising circumstances, there is an added level of trauma to consider when mourning the loss (Lichtenthal et al. 2010). After experiencing an existential crisis of meaning, how do bereaved mothers survive and find a reason to continue living? The following chapter will present the bereaved mother's journey of traumatic bereavement, and the key themes that reflect pertinent features of their traumatic loss.

Grief and Loss

When passing one's condolences or sympathy to a recently bereaved colleague, friend or family member, people often experience awkwardness and insufficient knowledge regarding the meaning of traumatic loss. The lack of clarity surrounding different types of bereavement is not helped by the controversy in the grief field in terms of the agreement of one clear definition of traumatic bereavement. Some grief experts believe traumatic bereavement belongs on a continuum theory of grief, viewing grief on a scale between 'normal', and 'complicated' or the possibility of experiencing pathological grief, which may require the diagnosis of a mental health disorder. However, medicalising grief is viewed as controversial in existential therapy, which avoids labelling and classifying a client's problems in living from a medical model (van Deurzen 2010). In spite of the evident confusion surrounding the difference between non-traumatic and traumatic loss, most grief experts agree that the experience of a sudden, unexpected death of a loved one is different to anticipatory loss and requires specialised knowledge and support in order to aid recovery (Glick et al. 1974; Parkes and Prigerson 2010; Worden 2009).

What Are the Features of Traumatic Bereavement?

Traumatic bereavement can be distinguished from a 'normal' bereavement based on several characteristics. The bereaved may experience a sense of powerlessness and helplessness, due to the sudden, unexpected death of a loved one, which can shatter the person's belief and trust in a benevolent and meaningful world that impacts their sense of control and safety (Herman 1992; Janoff-Bulman 1992; Kauffman 2002). In addition, it has been shown that grief lasts longer for bereaved parents, and they are more likely to face existential questions about the meaning and purpose of life, as they grapple with personal questions about their identity as a mother or parent (Wheeler 2001). Bereaved parents are a vulnerable bereavement population and are at greater risk of mortality, and from experiencing complex or complicated grief (Neimeyer et al. 2010; Parkes and Prigerson 2010; Young and Papadatou 1997). As a result, it is important to monitor bereaved parents closely in order to protect them from risk of harm.

The Importance of Being Heard

The bereaved mother's reasons for being interviewed were varied. However, they shared a similar motivation which reflected the need to help others, for example, by participating in traumatic bereavement research and sharing their personal perspectives. They believed that this type of activity would help clarify the confusion and misconceptions surrounding traumatic bereavement, in contrast to non-traumatic bereavement. Several bereaved mothers described the importance of having the opportunity to talk about their traumatic loss and their child, as they reflected that few people were willing, or were able to listen to the profoundly tragic experience of the death of a child, subsequent to the aftermath of the loss. Rose, who lost her 20-year-old son to suicide, described the overarching personal need to help others, and to campaign in the memory of her son to help raise awareness of the risks of suicide amongst young people. While for Violet, whose 18-year-old daughter also died by suicide, described being interviewed as cathartic, and also as an opportunity to talk freely about her daughter and how she died without being judged. The remaining bereaved mothers wanted to offer their perspective and stressed the lack of available information on the Internet. Some of the mothers also described the unhelpful procedures they had experienced at the hospital following the formal identification of their child's body. Nancy expressed her confusion regarding whether she could touch her daughter or hold her hand, after the fatal car accident which had killed her young adult daughter.

The Bereaved Mother's Stories: The Need to Be Kept Informed

Rose was informed of her son's death by the police, which she described as coming completely out of the blue. Although Rose had been aware of her son's prior mental health struggles, she was later personally tortured with guilt that her son had been suffering in silence, but could not share his despair with her. The inability to 'save' her son contributed to Rose's grief and suffering. Research has shown that guilt, shame and anger are common emotional responses following a death by suicide of a loved one (Wertheimer 2001).

The responsibility as a parent and mother to protect their child from pain and harm is emotionally challenged during the aftermath of a death by suicide. This triggers the unanswerable questions: 'Why couldn't I have stopped it?' and the innumerable 'what if' scenarios. Violet fantasised about what would have happened if she had noticed a missed call from her daughter shortly before she killed herself, torturing herself with the question, 'What if I hadn't gone into that meeting and seen her call?' The failure to foresee the unfathomable plays a role in the bereaved mother's parental guilt to protect their child from harm and pain, which can impact recovery from grief.

Ruth, whose 23-year-old son drowned, described wanting to understand the physiological process of drowning, and the need to know how long it would have taken her son to die, when he fatally slipped into a fast-moving river one wintry night on his way home. Her son was reported missing for a few days, and it was several weeks before the police found his body. The need to understand the final moments of their child's death and the degree to which they suffered was a common theme for the bereaved mothers.

Nancy viewed the post-mortem as another traumatic incident for her 26-year-old daughter and experienced the fact that they were going to cut into her daughter as invasive and traumatic. She would have preferred bereavement support from a grief counsellor or medical advisor who would explain the procedures. Ellen suffered the helplessness and sense of powerlessness that her daughter's death could have been prevented, if the GP had increased her daughter's epilepsy prescription on her last appointment. Ellen's daughter, Annie, who was 21, had been due to get married in six weeks; however, tragically she was buried in her wedding dress. Similar to Nancy's experience, Ellen wanted to protect her daughter from harm in death and was particularly disturbed that the post-mortem would leave a large visible scar.

For Sophie, who held strong religious beliefs, she suffered a dual trauma when she found her previously healthy 23-month-old toddler son dead on Christmas morning. The post-mortem revealed that her son had died from a viral strain of H1N1. Sophie wanted to be involved with all the official police and medical procedures, and as with the other mothers, she wanted to care for her child in death as she had in life. Sophie described wanting to hold the ruler when the police were required to take pictures of her son's body.

It is clear from the accounts of the bereaved mothers that they wanted and needed to be a part of their child's death in every aspect, from the procedural details to the post-mortem. This is an important and helpful response to trauma during the aftermath of the death of a child and impacts lifelong recovery from grief.

Isolating Experience: Absolute Separation from Others

The isolating experience is a ubiquitous grief response during bereavement. However, the traumatically bereaved mothers experienced a profound state of existential isolation, which is often precipitated after the confrontation with untimely death. Existential isolation refers to the individual's awareness of being completely and absolutely alone in the world, or as a separate *Being* from other people and the world (Yalom 1980). This type of isolation is also experienced when the individual becomes aware that they are the sole author of their life (Yalom 1980). This means that the awareness of the freedom to create and respond to one's suffering and existence reflects a powerful sense of aloneness and responsibility. The death of a child existentially isolated the bereaved mothers from other traumatically bereaved mothers, since it is only the individual who experiences the sense of aloneness and absolute separation from others that is unleashed after the sudden death of their child. Sophie described her experience of existential isolation poignantly:

> you can even be with other parents who have lost a child, but sometimes I feel lonely in that because [*pause*] of the kind of, unique, kind of circumstances around it, and that's a kind of isolation it's erm [*pause*] there might even be similarities around trauma [*pause*] but because of the complexities of it being swine flu and Christmas day, that kind of, it feels like we're kind of, you know, on an island by ourselves about that and that nobody else could, *possibly* kind of, you know, understand, or even relate to that.

The bereaved mothers experienced an estrangement from other people, as a result of the lack of knowledge and social stigma experienced in response to the tragic and horrifying circumstances surrounding their child's death. In addition, they experienced a sense of alienation and absolute separation from others as they described living outside the normal, everyday world following the loss of a child. However, the estrangement from others brings into stark reality the finding that the traumatically bereaved mothers were unable to return to the prior state of everyday living, which heightened the experience of isolation and alienation. This was due to a loss of innocence in the prior trust and belief in a fair and meaningful existence. Although the mothers experienced a new way of *Being-in-the-world*, the gap between them and the non-traumatically bereaved widens, which contributed to the sense of existential isolation and alienation. Ellen described her vulnerability and the need to wear a badge that identified her as having experienced a horrible tragedy:

> I almost feel like I need to walk around with a badge, you know let people know I'm not the same as you, you know, I'm, it's like with people who've had this kind of death, it's almost like you feel outside of society you know, it's almost like you feel, I feel, separate.

Ellen's description of wearing a visual marker that connects her to the traumatically bereaved highlights the longing to belong and connect with others. However, the suggestion of wearing a badge intensifies the estrangement and alienation from others, and there is a danger that the bereaved mothers may further isolate themselves from potential connections, or remain with their in-group—the traumatically bereaved.

The death of a child clarifies other parent's greatest fear, which they may be unwilling to consider (Doka 2002; Gorer 1987; Young and Papadatou 1997). The bereaved mothers experienced social exclusion and stigma, which potentially reflects the heightened death taboo surrounding society's reluctance, and specifically other parent's reluctance to consider the potential death of their child (Walter 2017). Ruth described the overt unwillingness of a young woman she met on the beach one day, to engage with death and her loss. As the young woman saw Ruth approaching, she ran away in horror clutching her young child. Ruth reflected that the terror of death was experienced as though you 'could catch death, as though it was contagious'.

The tragedy, horror and sometimes violent circumstances surrounding their child's death alienated the bereaved mothers from others, for example, Nancy described experiencing the divisive impact of telling people her daughter was killed, in contrast to saying that her daughter had died. She noticed the impact of explaining the violent circumstances of her daughter's death and observed how people visibly withdrew from the conversation, saying:

> I notice that if I use the word killed, if I say, erm, my daughter was killed, there's I, I can feel the tension in the other person…it's hard it's like you shock them and you can tell that they don't reach out for you the same way, they become sort of like it's almost like they stand back and it's like they then don't know what to say next.

This theme is paradoxical because the lack of social awareness and knowledge about the lived experience of traumatic bereavement perpetuates the isolating experience for the bereaved mothers. The experience of insensitive and damaging responses to their loss increased a sense of self-isolation because the bereaved mothers were reluctant to interact with those who increased their pain and suffering. In the twenty-first century, in Western society people are unwilling to engage with the taboo subject of death, and view death procedures as morbid. As a result, people often avoid thinking about death, and the death of loved ones until they come face to face with death, which is an inevitable given of the human condition. However, when the death is tragic, violent, and frightening many people are shocked, and experience discomfort, which contributes to the bereaved mother's experience of estrangement and alienation from others.

Self-Protection: Wearing an Inauthentic Grief Mask

As a result of the damaging and insensitive response to their loss, the traumatically bereaved mothers distanced themselves from others, and normalised their traumatic grief response through changing the shocking details of the death and devising a story that they felt comfortable sharing with others. This helped reduce the personal impact of coping with the insensitive response to the loss. The mothers emotionally self-protect by compartmentalising their private grief journey and monitoring the degree they reveal their traumatic loss to others. This grief response enabled the mothers to cope with other people's discomfort when faced with the reality of a sudden, violent loss of a child and in some cases the stigmatisation of the loss. The mothers felt responsible for managing the direction of the conversation while talking about their loss and were mindful of the personal consequences of coping with other people's discomfort and shock. Rose described her experience of this:

> it's not easy when you tell somebody, it's horrible on them and every time I told somebody I was reminded of when I was told and how horrible that was so that stopped me actually from telling other people because I was like they're going to be shocked, I was trying to protect them.

The bereaved mothers experienced concern that other people would perceive them differently, which reflects a paradox. On the one hand, they longed to share their loss with others, and talk openly about their child. However, on the other hand, they were reluctant to be identified as the 'traumatically bereaved mother' or having experienced a terrible loss. Violet worked hard to conceal the truth and pain of her loss, saying 'I've worked at this, I don't want people looking at me and thinking I can see that she's suffered a tremendous loss, I don't want to invoke pity, so I almost work at being normal'.

This reflects a development in the self-protection recovery process, as the mothers move from the vulnerable state of self-protection, wishing to tell everybody about their painful and horrible loss, to the state where they feel comfortable sharing aspects of their loss, yet keeping their ongoing personal grief private. Sophie described her experience of this poignantly 'I used to kind of lay it on with a trowel, yes my child died, yes it was like a cot death oh and by the way it happened on Christmas Day'. Yet as time passed, she did not feel the need to share all the shocking details of her loss.

The self-protection theme served a purpose for the bereaved mothers, which helped them to emotionally and socially self-protect from traumatic overload in the everyday ontic world during their vulnerable psychological state. The Western sociocultural attitude towards death and mourning, and the impact of the death taboo influenced the bereaved mother's social adaptation to grief and the loss of a child. Macquarrie

(1972) wrote extensively about Heidegger's (1962) existential theories of existence. Heidegger (1962) believed that death is the ultimate future possibility for the 'Dasein', which refers to the concept that the individual exists in a context of the world. Heidegger proposed that human existence is defined by the human given of *not* being. It is inevitable that death will occur at some unknown point in the future. In other words, the human being is determined by their awareness of mortality and exists as a *Being towards-death*. Heidegger (1962) argued that if the individual is aware of the human given of *not* being, or the finitude of existence, they may struggle with the state of caring about the world, caring about others or themselves and living a meaningful life—creating an ongoing tension between caring for the world and others which is potentially intensified or diminished. However, an awareness of existence in the face of their ultimate demise can inspire an individual to live purposefully and strive for meaning.

Macquarrie proposed that the bereaved individual needs to fit in with 'Das Man' or the masses regarding sociocultural expectations surrounding death and mourning, which he compared to Western society's 'flight and avoidance' (Macquarrie 1972: 197) attitude towards death, and that 'it will be business as usual' (ibid.: 198) post loss. However, wearing an inauthentic grief mask and normalising the traumatic grief response isolates the bereaved mothers from potential help and support. The inauthentic grief mask refers to the difficulty the bereaved mothers experienced sharing the distressing aspects of grief with loved ones, friends and colleagues, for example, sharing feelings of not being able to cope, experiencing panic attacks, nightmares, anxiety, depression and experiencing suicidal thoughts (Pitman et al. 2018). As a result, the mothers normalised their grief response in social situations, in order to conceal the reality of their experience.

Ongoing Bond with Loved One

The ongoing bond theme is an important part of the traumatically bereaved mother's journey to recovery. The ongoing bond reflects the significance of maintaining a relationship with the deceased child that brings meaning and comfort to the bereaved mother. Sophie summarised the importance of this bond in the quote at the beginning of this chapter, in other words, just because her child is dead it does not mean she does not have a continuing spiritual[1] or personal relationship with her child. The ongoing bond grief literature is vast and has highlighted the progress in knowledge from traditional grief models that proposed recovery from grief occurs when the attachment bond to the loved one is severed, and the bereaved 'moves on' from the loss (Freud 1957; Worden 2009). However, the ongoing bonds model of grief recognises that a continuing relationship with the loved one supports healing and recovery from loss (Klass et al. 1996; Klass and Steffen 2018).

The bereaved mothers recognised the difference between continuing to mourn the pain and sorrow for the loss of their child and developing an ongoing relationship. For some this was a spiritual connection, in terms of gaining comfort from a religious belief that was strengthened post loss. Sophie, for example, believed that her child was being held by the religious mother figure Mary, which brought her relief and comfort. However, for others, a lack of religious belief was comforting. Ruth reflected feeling relieved that her son was not aware of the reality he was missing out on:

> I think I would find it absolutely unbearable if I had a faith, if I had some idea sense of an afterlife kind of traditional Christian...you know, sort of, rather woolly traditional Christianity I was brought up in of heaven and people being able to look down, and angels in the sky and all that, erm how fucking awful that he could see this, that he would know what he's missing and see [*crying*] and see me this broken.

The ongoing bond with their child supported the bereaved mother's process of identifying new meaning in their lives, without feeling guilty that they were 'forgetting' their child or honouring their memory if they rebuild meaning. For example, four years post loss, Nancy described the ongoing struggle to separate her belief that she was being disloyal to her daughter if she goes on to pursue meaning. Nancy's experience highlights

[1]Spiritual relationship refers to an existential understanding of the spiritual dimension (for a fuller description, see Chapters 2 and 15).

the importance for some bereaved mothers, to identify meaning making with the memory of the loved one. Sophie now works with bereaved children or pre-bereavement which brings meaning to her life and enables her to feel connected to her son, while Violet and Rose described the importance of maintaining an ongoing bond with their children from the activities they pursue, for example, campaigning for suicide awareness.

The ongoing bond develops and changes with time, some bereaved mothers acknowledged the importance of separating their continuing bond from the pain and sorrow of their loss. However, it is a complex process, which is interwoven, as Ruth highlighted 'somehow it's about holding Jack, it's not about thinking lovely memories and happy things and putting him in that sort of memorialising box'. The ongoing bond brings comfort and meaning to the bereaved mothers, which helps them move forward in their journey, and have the courage to rebuild and pursue meaning.

Embodied Response: Ongoing Sorrow

> Of course I'm broken I think there's something that represents the strength of my love for my son why the hell would I not be broken, why would I just be a bit bruised? (Ruth)

This is an important finding for the bereaved mothers, since it reflects the relationship between their psychological grief response to their physical changes and the management of these changes. The mothers used a variety of expressions to describe the physical impact of the loss on the body, ranging from 'physical illness', 'cold tar', the 'heaviness' or the 'weight' of grief and feeling 'broken'. The physical manifestation of grief impacted the bereaved mother's resilience to cope with daily life and highlighted their concerns that the physical changes will be ongoing. Nancy described the impact of experiencing a depressed mood on her outlook of life 'I don't feel as if there's that light airiness about me that there used to be, everything feels closed in and crowded', while Ruth described the physical response as dragging around the feeling of heaviness of her body. The sense of feeling broken was not viewed as a negative experience of the mother's traumatic loss, but as a reflection of their profound loss. The mothers viewed their emotional 'brokenness' as a symbol of their ongoing love and pain for the loss of their child.

Although it becomes easier with time for the traumatically bereaved mothers to manage their raw grief, the visceral pain does resurface. Violet said 'in a way I lock it away, one, so I can put on this public face and two, appear as an amazing brave person carrying off life, and three, to save myself from myself because if I feel like if I gave into it, and allowed it free reign I would just walk in front of a train'. This process reflects the bereaved mother's psychological growth which enables them to self-protect from the pain and sorrow of grief. However, they acknowledged that ongoing sorrow is now part of their continued existence.

Loss of Meaning: Frozen Future

The traumatically bereaved mothers experienced a lack of safety in the world, which impacted their psychological ability to trust and plan for the future, which was termed 'frozen future'. The mothers experienced the future as unimaginable and full of uncertainty. The sudden confrontation with the loss of a child triggered the bereaved mother's experience of existential anxiety, which is a response to the awakening of the uncertainty or underlying 'Angst' (May 1977: 210) or unease that accompanies the awareness that their existence is beyond the comfort and safety of the everyday world (van Deurzen 2002). This type of anxiety confronts the individual with the fear of the very real possibility of one's demise, and potential free fall into the abyss of despair alongside the meaninglessness of existence. However, an individual has the freedom to choose from the limitless possibilities of existence, which is experienced as an overwhelming responsibility that is referred to as existential anxiety (see May 1977; Sartre 1957). The experience of this type of anxiety for the bereaved mothers can be described as an existential crisis of motherhood. In other words, the bereaved mothers experienced a sudden awareness of the lack of control in life, which raised existential anxiety about the safety of the world, and the mortality of loved ones. Ellen described her increased fear of existence:

> It's just scary really, life is scary now in a way that it wasn't before you know… I'm forever anxious about something else happening, you know, fear of [*sighs*] I don't know of losing things that I love… Yeah it's like the safety net's gone that's the thing you know, that's what Annie's death has done it's taken away the safety net.

For some, the confrontation with despair and suffering raised existential questions about the meaning and purpose of life. It impacted their appreciation for spending time with significant people in their lives, and valuing meaningful connections with others, which brings comfort, healing and happiness into their lives. The questioning of existence and the meaning of life were particularly strong for the mothers who lost an only child. Violet described experiencing a total obliteration of her identity as a mother and parent, which left her questioning her purpose and meaning in life. She struggled with the questions, 'Why am I here?' and 'What's the point?' because a large part of her existence had been focused on looking after her daughter and meeting her needs:

> it was, you know a complete um wipe out of everything that had defined me before, um because Rose was the, was an only child so it was suddenly a you know home without a child in it…a whole existence before had centred around being her life support if you like, making sure she had clean clothes and money, and was safe and didn't get in too late and didn't wear too much make-up and all of that wiped out, so you suddenly think wha-well what's the, why am I here, you know what's the point.

The bereaved mothers found the courage and inner strength (or resilience[2]) to survive the unimaginable pain of the loss of a child. Ruth described her certainty that before the loss of her son if one of her children had died she would die, however, post loss, she was surprised that

[2]In this context, resilience does not refer to the perspective of thriving from adversity, as in the posttraumatic growth literature, but to psychological growth or 'strength' (Calhoun et al. 2010).

she was 'still standing'. Although Violet described her daughter's decision to end her life as courageous and determined, she expressed her continual daily struggle to choose life, and not act on her own suicidal thoughts. The existential philosopher, Camus (1955) posed the question, 'Is life worth living or would one be better off killing themselves?' He believed that the philosophical question regarding the absurdity of life could be answered by living a meaningful life, Camus (1955) suggested that the absurdity of life begins with the repetition of daily life, which represents the potential meaninglessness of existence. However, the meaninglessness of life is replaced when the individual chooses a life filled with meaning and purpose. For Violet, although she experienced the meaninglessness of life and questioned her existence and purpose without her daughter, she chose to embrace life, take on new challenges and find a different purpose:

> you know all meaning was taken away really with Rose dying and um, and all those statuses going you know, the mother, parent [*pause*] so what brings meaning now [*long pause*] I don't know if it's the same thing but you know, I have wh-what's what is it that I couldn't live without now, or what kind of life have I built for myself, I've built one where um, activity's very important, so I run and I train for things and that gives me a goal, so it will be a half marathon this year, I run for 'P' which is a charity [that] supports er prevention of young suicide, um I do certain things so that Rose's remembered, so, um, I have a tree in the park.

The loss of meaning theme reflects the existential paradox of the absurdity and meaninglessness of existence, while highlighting the importance of the individual taking responsibility for identifying a daily purpose and finding meaning in one's life.

The prior trust and belief in a fair and meaningful existence filled with hopes and dreams for their children's future have been permanently shattered, and a personal worldview about the natural order of life obliterated. In order to cope with the fear and existential anxiety about the uncertainty and unpredictability of a now unsafe world, and the anxiety surrounding the possibility of remaining in despair, the bereaved mothers developed emotional coping strategies, which brought temporary comfort and solace. This was observed in their ambivalent feelings about the future, and the reluctance to commit to future plans based on the belief 'We might not be here', or as Violet reflected 'If I don't dream I won't be let down and hurt again'. The duration since the loss impacted the experience of loss of meaning and a frozen future, for example, Sophie, who experienced her loss 7 years ago, was able to imagine a future, and described it as 'hopeful'. However, the mothers, who experienced their loss between 1.5 and 4 years ago, expressed difficulties planning for the future, or the reluctance to embrace the pursuit of personal hopes and dreams. The bereaved mother's difficulties to imagine and plan for the future can impact meaning making, which is an important part of adaptation to loss, and subsequent healing.

Pursuit of Meaning: Being with Others

The pursuit of meaning highlights the bereaved mother's experience of finding a way to survive in the face of loss and despair. This was identified from the pursuit of personally meaningful activities and relationships. Meaning making is a complex process for the bereaved mothers, and some mothers did not identify a personally meaningful purpose. This reflects the psychological risk that bereaved mothers can experience complicated grief and remain frozen in grief, when they are unable to separate their ongoing grief and sorrow from rebuilding meaning. For Ellen, three years post loss, she experienced the reconstruction of meaning as elusive, and described being unable to comprehend how she is surviving:

> it's hard work to stay alive you know I've been on anti-depressants for pretty much, well probably, a few months after she died um and I have huge lows you know, I, there are still times when I don't want to carry on, I'm not, I'm not suicidal I wouldn't do anything about it but there are still a lot of times that I don't want to be here if, if I didn't have other children I wouldn't be here you know at all.

Ellen's struggle to identify personal meaning, aside from caring for her other children, highlights how subsequent recovery is impacted by complex trauma and that psychological growth is required in order to move forward from this acute state of grief, and avoid remaining frozen in hopelessness and despair.

The bereaved mothers recognised the importance of developing and nurturing meaningful relationships with others, which reflects the human need for love and care, and is an important part of recovery from traumatic bereavement. Meaningful connections provided support and friendship and allowed the bereaved mothers to grieve naturally. This was a highly valued experience in the mother's recovery, which despite the sociocultural expectations surrounding grief and mourning, prompted them to normalise grief. However, the range of emotional responses during traumatic grief, including, humour and laughter, and the capacity to 'let off steam' was also considered an important aspect of the development of supportive connections with others traumatically bereaved. Ruth described the emotional freedom she experienced with a friend whose young adult daughter had died:

> we can say the unsayable and we can also say the funny things and the black things and be inappropriate and you know just maybe the opposite of the erm grieving with the vapors, we can also be sassy and funny and grumpy and angry and all the emotions that are perhaps not associated with society's idea of grief.

This theme reflects the importance of social contact in healing and recovery from grief, and the value of gaining emotional support from friends, and developing meaningful connections with others. This reflects Heidegger's (1962) concept of solicitude, which proposes that human beings are motivated to coexist with others based on the human need to be cared for, to care for others or to care about a particular aspect of the world. This is based on the existential theory of Being-*in*-the-world. In other words, the bereaved mothers cannot avoid existing *in* relation to the world and *in* relation to others in their everyday lives, and the development of meaningful relationships supports their journey through the unimaginable pain of losing a child.

The meaningful relationships theme provided support and comfort from two perspectives, one, this encouraged the mothers to grieve openly, and two, it increased an appreciation for the value of meaningful dialogue, and the significance of investing time and energy in relationships. Rose reflected 'we can't give anything anybody but our time…if we can't give each other time and attention and compassion then erhm we have nothing to give to each other'. The pursuit of a meaning-based existence filled with meaningful connections reflects the importance of nurturing relationships that provide safety, support and friendship, and for some the opportunity to grieve without the grief mask. This is an important theme because it reduces the isolating experience and the bereaved mother's need to self-protect during traumatic grief, which isolates them from potential help and support.

Conclusion

The psychological growth that enables the bereaved mothers to begin the process of identifying and rebuilding personal meaning reflects the acknowledgement of a gradual separation from the primary identity as a traumatically bereaved mother and a daily existence filled with acute grief and suffering (there is no time frame for this), and the new emerging identity that encompasses the profound loss of a child as part of their ongoing existence. The frequently used metaphor 'emotional scar of loss' (Wertheimer 2001) is an apt description for the transition between the acute experience of traumatic grief and being psychologically vulnerable, and the gradual reluctance to be solely defined by profound and tragic loss.

It is important to acknowledge the paradox seen in the bereaved mother's experience of traumatic bereavement, which on the one hand reflects personal growth or resilience, and the courage to survive the unimaginable loss of a child. This was seen in the arduous and painful journey through meaninglessness and adversity, in order to reach a state that enabled the possibility of rebuilding a meaningful existence, for example, helping others through suffering, campaigning in their child's memory, and valuing friendships. However, on the other hand, the traumatically bereaved mothers continue to exist with their ongoing sorrow and physical changes, which reflects their love and pain for the loss of their child. As time passes, the bereaved mothers integrate their sorrow and raw grief into their daily existence, and learn to monitor the degree they 'go into the black' as Ruth described. The development of the ongoing bond supports the lifelong journey of ongoing sorrow, which diminishes with time, but as Sophie described the grief is just below the surface, and a scratch can trigger the raw pain and despair for a mother's traumatic loss of a child.

References

Bowlby, J. (1980). *Attachment and Loss, Volume 3: Loss, Sadness and Depression.* Middlesex, UK: Penguin Books.

Calhoun, L. G., Tedeschi, R. G., Cann, A., & Hanks, E. A. (2010). Positive Outcomes Following Bereavement: Paths to Posttraumatic Growth. *Psychologica Belgica, 50*(1–2), 125–143.

Camus, A. (1942/1955). *The Myth of Sisyphus* (J. O'Brian, Trans.). London: Penguin Books Ltd.

Doka, K. J. (2002). How We Die: Stigmatized Death and Disenfranchised Grief. In K. J. Doka (Ed.), *Disenfranchised Grief: New Directions, Challenges, and Strategies for Practice*. Champaign, IL: Research Press.

Freud, S. (1917/1957). Mourning and Melancholia. In J. Strachey (Ed.), *The Standard Edition of the Complete Psychological Works of Sigmund Freud Volume XIV (vol. 14).* London: Hogarth Press and The Institute of Psycho-Analysis.

Glick, I. O., Weiss, R. S., & Parkes, C. M. (1974). *The First Year of Bereavement*. New York, NY: Wiley.

Gorer, G. (1987). *Death, Grief, and Mourning in Contemporary Britain.* Salem, New Hampshire: Ayer.

Heidegger, M. (1927/1962). *Being and Time* (J. Macquarrie & E. S. Robinson, Trans.). Malden, MA and Oxford: Blackwell.

Herman, J. (1992). *Trauma and Recovery.* New York, NY: Basic Books.

Janoff-Bulman, R. (1992). *Shattered Assumptions Towards a New Psychology of Trauma.* New York, NY: The Free Press.

Kauffman, J. (2002). Safety and the Assumptive World. In J. Kauffman (Ed.), *Loss of the Assumptive World: A Theory of Assumptive Loss.* New York, NY and London: Brunner-Routledge.

Klass, D., Silverman, P. R., & Nickman, S. L. (Eds.). (1996). *Continuing Bonds: New Understandings of Grief*. Washington, DC: Taylor & Francis.

Klass, D., & Steffen, E. M. (Eds.). (2018). *Continuing Bonds in Bereavement: New Directions for Research and Practice*. New York, NY: Routledge.

Lichtenthal, W. G., Currier, J. M., Neimeyer, R. A., & Keesee, N. J. (2010). Sense and Significance. A Mixed Methods Examination of Meaning Making After the Loss of One's Child. *Journal of Clinical Psychology, 66*(7), 791–812. https://doi.org/10.1002/jclp.20700.

Macquarrie, J. (1972). *Existentialism*. London: Penguin Books.

May, R. (1977). *The Meaning of Anxiety*. New York, NY: W. W. Norton.

McClowry, S. G., Davies, E. B., May, K. A., Kulenkamp, E. J., & Martinson, I. M. (1987). The Empty Space Phenomenon: The Process of Grief in the Bereaved Family. *Death Studies, 11*(5), 361–374. https://doi.org/10.1080/07481188708252200.

Neimeyer, R. A., Burke, L. A., Mackay, M. M., & van Dyke Stringer, J. G. (2010). Grief Therapy and the Reconstruction of Meaning: From Principles to Practice. *Journal of Contemporary Psychotherapy, 40*(2), 73–83.

Parkes, C. M., & Prigerson, H. G. (2010). *Bereavement Studies of Grief in Adult Life* (4th ed.). London: Penguin Books.

Pitman, A. L., Stevenson, F., Osborn, D. P. J., & King, M. B. (2018). The Stigma Associated with Bereavement by Suicide and Other Sudden Deaths: A Qualitative Study. *Social Science & Medicine, 198*, 121–129. https://doi.org/10.1016/j.socscimed.2017.12.035.

Rando, T. A. (1993). *Treatment of Complicated Mourning*. Champaign, IL: Research Press.

Rynearson, E. K., Schut, H., & Stroebe, M. (2013). Complicated Grief After Violent Death: Identification and Intervention. In M. Stroebe, H. Schut, & J. van den Bout (Eds.), *Complicated Grief: Scientific Foundations for Health Care Professionals*. Hove, East Sussex: Routledge.

Sartre, J.-P. (1943/1957). *Being and Nothingness: An Essay on Phenomenological Ontology* (H. E. Barnes, Trans.). London: Methuen & Co Ltd.

Seigal, C. (2017). *Bereaved Parents and their Continuing Bonds: Love After Death*. London: Jessica Kingsley Publishers.

van Deurzen, E. (2002). *Existential Counselling and Psychotherapy in Practice* (2nd ed.). London: Sage.

van Deurzen, E. (2010). *Everyday Mysteries, a Handbook of Existential Psychotherapy* (2nd ed.). Hove, East Sussex: Routledge.

Walter, T. (2017). *What Death Means Now: Thinking Critically About Dying and Grieving*. Bristol: Policy Press.

Wertheimer, A. (2001). *A Special Scar: The Experiences of People Bereaved by Suicide* (2nd ed.). Hove, East Sussex: Brunner-Routledge.

Wheeler, I. (2001). Parental Bereavement: The Crisis of Meaning. *Death Studies, 25*(1), 51–66.

Worden, J. W. (2009). *Grief Counselling and Grief Therapy: A Handbook for the Mental Health Practitioner* (4th ed.). London and New York, NY: Routledge.

Yalom, I. D. (1980). *Existential Psychotherapy*. New York, NY: Basic Books.

Young, B., & Papadatou, D. (1997). Childhood, Death and Bereavement Across Cultures. In C. M. Parkes, P. Laungani, & B. Young (Eds.), *Death and Bereavement Across Cultures*. London and New York, NY: Routledge.

12

Trying to "Have-It-All" at 30; Timing Motherhood

Naomi Magnus

> I believe increasingly that only the willingness to share private and sometimes painful experience can enable women to create a collective description of the world which will be truly ours. (Rich 1986: 16)

Existential Considerations

In his introduction to *Being and Time* (1927), Heidegger proposed that *time* is the context or horizon against which Being is revealed, and therefore, Being must be grasped "*in terms of time*: our sense of what it is to be must depend on temporality" (Polt 1999: 25). According to Heidegger, fundamentally humans are temporal, meaning we exist in time and in the process of existing, Being is revealed (Heidegger 1927). In existential philosophy, the term *temporality* is used to denote the way in which time exists and is experienced in human existence (Warnock 1970: 62). In addition, it is not just that as humans we experience time, but that

N. Magnus (✉)
UKCP, London, UK

C. Arnold-Baker (ed.), *The Existential Crisis of Motherhood*,
https://doi.org/10.1007/978-3-030-56499-5_12

we *care* about, and are concerned with our existence and hence the time that we experience: "temporality and care qualify human existence" (Weixel-Dixon and Strasser 2005: 230).

Heidegger's phenomenology of time understands time as a phenomenon to be experienced as other phenomena. For Heidegger, the counting and measuring of time of Aristotle and the conception of it as a sequence of "nows", which lead to distinct time dimensions, are false constructs that come out of humans' inherent need to compartmentalise and therefore attempt to understand existence, but it does not tell us anything about time itself and our relationship to it (Cohn 2002: 63). Instead, Heidegger proposed a conception of time where "there is no linear move from past via present to future, as every present moment still contains the past it left behind while already pointing towards the future" (ibid.: 64). Therefore, Dasein's experience of the present moment will always contain elements of its past and future, a temporality that sets it apart from other existing things, this experience of time is uniquely human.

Indeed, for Heidegger our temporality is "ecstatical", we stand-out (Polt 1999: 97), as opposed to present-at-hand entities, with a definite past and present, we have the ability to transcend our immediate situation, meaning we are able to be in a present that contains the past and points towards the future (Cohn 2002: 66). For Heidegger, our openness to and awareness of our ability to transcend time, and the presence of time as a backdrop to our lives is authentic living: "in inauthenticity, the past and future are *subordinated* to the present, whereas in authenticity the present gains a fresh and deeper meaning from the past, and especially, from the future" (Polt 1999: 100).

For humans time is always finite, it comes to an end with our death. If authentic existence is an openness to and acceptance of the way in which time exists for Dasein, to live authentically we must constantly project our lives onto the horizon of our death, living with a profound understanding of our inevitable finitude, Heidegger terms this "being-towards-death" (Heidegger 1927). Indeed, time only exists for us from a mortal vantage point, time has meaning for us through our finitude. For Heidegger, my mortality is my "ownmost" possibility (ibid.), it is my own, I cannot die someone else's death or escape my own, and it is this that gives my life meaning, as with death, my life is mine to live, I cannot live another (Polt 1999: 87). Heidegger proposes that authentic living is a way of being in which Dasein is truly itself, when we are not absorbed in the they-self but instead live with integrity and clarity and an awareness of the "givens" of existence, it requires "facing up to mortality - not by worrying about when demise will come, but by accepting the finitude of one's possibilities and choosing in the light of this finitude" (ibid.).

Jaspers (1951) emphasised "limit situations", situations that enhance our awareness of this finitude and our finality and may create angst that when explored reveal our relationship to our mortality. Circumstances such as ending a psychotherapeutic relationship act as "limit situations" and may bring a person closer to their authentic response to their own mortality and existence.

On beginning my studies in existential psychotherapy, it struck me that there was little to no writing on the finitude of fertility as one of the *existentials* or givens of existence for women. I wondered whether the uncertainty around the finitude of our fertility acted as a limit situation (Jaspers 1951) for women who want children, and in turn meant that we were confronted with our mortality and temporality earlier than our male counterparts. The anxiety that I was feeling around my fertility reflected much of my anxieties connected to my life as a whole, such as feeling an ever-present awareness of limited time and anxiety around my limits in a larger sense.

Women's experiences of life and living have been notably neglected by much of the existential literature. Academically, the "biological clock" has been researched to date mostly from more practical perspectives—investigations into egg freezing, single mothers by choice, balancing a career and motherhood and other such topics abound (e.g. Dillaway and Pare 2008; Raspberry and Skinner 2011), yet little has been said about how women who want children experience their lives as a whole against the backdrop of their finite fertility.

Approaching my thirties, as a woman who wants to have children, I began to feel a growing sense of urgency towards my existence. I was raised in a middle-class, educated family and community, sent to an academically competitive private girls' school, and encouraged to consider what I wanted to "do" for as long as I can remember. Raised by a mother who was influenced by the feminism of the seventies (e.g. Greer 1970), I was encouraged to think about a career in exactly the same way that my brother was, I was not told that as a woman, my life trajectory and priorities may look different to my brother's. I knew I wanted a family, but I was not guided to think strategically about this part of my life, it seemed taken as a given that it would just fit in somewhere. Turning thirty, with other priorities filling my life, I became increasingly aware of the finitude of my fertility, as I found myself narrowing the window of opportunity I had to conceive. This narrowing window gave rise to a consciousness of the specific experience of timing motherhood. The thoughts and feelings I had around choosing when to mother were inextricably linked to a felt sense of the finitude of my fertility alongside my life trajectory and decisions, specifically around my career.

I was inspired to think further about this specific and unique phenomenon, how do other women experience it? Are there common parts of the experience? Can a deeper understanding of the phenomenon of timing motherhood alongside career planning and age 30 in some way provide a new awareness and proficiency for existential practitioners?

Through personal exploration and a semi-structured conversation with a woman in a similar circumstance, I set out to explore and illuminate how professional women experience desiring to mother and career planning against the backdrop of the finitude of their fertility. This experience is explored in a specific context of geography and time, and therefore, I will first set the scene and situate the experience and the main themes.

Women as Wives and Mothers

Female identity has long been linked with the notion of mothering and reproduction. Stories involving female characters in religious texts such as the Old Testament often focus on them as mothers or not mothers, with those who are fertile and able to carry future generations in their wombs triumphing while the barren are pitied (Zornberg 2009). Consequently, female narratives in such texts are reduced to their biology and their ability or inability to mother, with other facets of their characters of little interest or relevance. As such, the inherited latent narrative for women seemed to be that we are mothers or not mothers and any other realm of female lived experience is of little or no consequence.

Such a stance persisted into the twentieth century, bolstered by Freud and the popularity of psychoanalysis, which further connected woman to her biology and fertility. Freud's theories of female sexuality ultimately led to the notion that "normal" development resulted in heterosexual girls becoming mothers. Psychoanalytic ideas of female sexuality and neuroses begin with the notion that upon reaching the oedipal stage little girls became aware of their fundamental lack and positioning as lesser as compared to boys (Freud 1905). Freud's assertion was that women mature to seek sexual pleasure through heterosexual vaginal intercourse, as grown-up women "should" experience an urge towards motherhood, finding compensation for lacking a penis through having children. In a similar vein, Medard Boss, in his book *The Meaning and Content of Sexual Perversions* (Boss and Diethelm 1949) wrote about "homosexuality as a sexual perversion" and in 1987 stated that "the healthiest state for a woman was to have children in a loving relationship with a man" (cited in Langdridge and Barker 2013: 148).

De Beauvoir wrote: in adolescence: "woman learns that for her there is to be no conquest, that she must disown herself, that her future depends upon man's good pleasure" (de Beauvoir 1949: 382). Societies inherited expectations of women was that they were to be tethered to a male and subsequently reproduce and mother in order to be considered "adult". This expectation created a status quo in Western societies where "normal" female development resulted in wifedom and motherhood. Rich suggests that the patriarchy created a society of "compulsory heterosexuality" (Rich 1980: 637) where heterosexuality maintains the status quo acting to keep women dependent on men, and accepting of their lot as wife-and-mothers.

Accordingly, motherhood and monogamous, heterosexual coupledom have become intertwined with understandings of female sexuality, and any sense that sexuality exists in females outside of these norms has seldom been considered. Correspondingly, heterosexuality has persisted as "normal" sexuality, and mothering as inherently connected to the female expression of sexuality and adult female experience. Such a feeling endures in Western societies such as the UK, where "heteronormative" or "pronatalist" societies continue to perpetuate the notion that having children is a natural and inevitable part of being a woman (Rowland 1992) and position women who are not heterosexual mothers outside of the "norm" (Jackson 2006). Hence, the idea that women are mothers and becoming a mother in some way fulfils an inevitable destiny prevails, with many women seeing motherhood as an inevitable part of their adult life.

Indeed, in Jacques and Radtke's (2012) study they showed that young heterosexual Canadian women, educated to degree level, continue to project their future life trajectories along traditional notions of womanhood as wife-and-mother (Jacques and Radtke 2012). Correspondingly, Segal et al. (2001) found that 100% of female college students anticipated that they would marry in the future and 96% anticipated having children. As such, it would seem that while women in the twenty-first century have more varied choice in terms of life trajectory, motherhood remains a given for the majority.

The academic community has largely neglected women's lived experience of existing within Western, pronatalist societies, instead focusing on more biological aspects of fertility and studies that look at what young women are "doing" rather than "experiencing".

The Significance of Thirty

Although ideas vary around when is the time to "panic" regarding fertility, there is general consensus that the older we are the harder it is to conceive. While an increasing number of women are planning motherhood in their mid-to-late thirties, ageing continues to be associated with compromised ovarian function and decreasing fecundity (Baird et al. 2005; Korula and Mohan 2010; Madankumar et al. 2003). Indeed, fertility in women is known to decline after the age of 30, strikingly so after 35 (Navot and Bergh 1991), as such biologically, there *is* cause for increased urgency regarding motherhood at age thirty. Klay (2009) proposes that statistics such as these are increasingly significant in the twenty-first century since more women in their middle-to-late 20s are developing the self through career and education and delaying reproduction until their 30s.

As such, there seems to be increased anxiety around the desire to mother in women specifically approaching and turning thirty (Macko and Rubin 2004). Macko and Rubin (2004) propose the emergence of a "midlife crisis at 30" for women of the X/Y generation. Data shows that "today's young women are getting married, having babies, and making major decisions about the directions of their careers at a very compressed juncture – right around their thirtieth birthdays" (ibid.: 3). Consequently, it seems that increased pressure around this time to have each different parts of their lives "sorted" leads young women to question "what's wrong with us" when they don't (ibid.). With women's role in Western society continuing to shift, Klay advocates that symptoms associated with this increased pressure such as anxiety and stress must be acknowledged and recognised, not only in the field of psychology but also in the larger culture, in order to help decrease the symptoms and "normalize" the experience (Klay 2009).

Culturally shared narratives regarding female life course and motherhood prevail in Western countries (Chodorow and Contratto 1992; Meyers 2001); it seems that at the level of cultural narrative there is a very narrow right time to become a mother. It would appear that these narratives adjust the thinking of women to consider the correct time to become a mother in relation to the right age at which it is permissible and, furthermore, to the right moment in the life course, e.g. only when at a certain career point (Woollett and Boyle 2000).

While models that saw anatomy as destiny for women have been cast aside with an acknowledgement that they have little to offer to the discussion in contemporary Western society, anatomy and finite fertility remain a given for women. Fertility is finite and this is something that we are more aware of in the modern world where we have choices and roles other than motherhood that may fill the years that we have to conceive.

Having-It-All

The approval of the combined oral contraceptive pill in the United States in 1960 made it easier for women to have careers by being able to control *when* and *if* they had children (Tone 2001). Indeed, the availability of the pill in 1961 is often credited as a catalyst in making a second wave of feminism possible, a wave that mostly focused on getting women out of the home and into the workplace (ibid.).

In 1963 Betty Friedan, influenced by de Beauvoir's *The Second Sex* (1949), wrote her seminal book *The Feminine Mystique* which is credited as kick-starting this new wave. In her book, Friedan suggested that "occupation: housewife" placed women at home, limiting them and their possibilities. Instead, she advocated access to higher levels of education for women, showing through a survey she conducted that women who played roles in the workforce and at home concurrently were more satisfied with life as compared to those who were "sad and agitated" by being housewives only (Friedan 2001).

This specific wave of feminism made space for new conversations around how women could juggle motherhood and working life at the same time while succeeding at both. Such a notion became encapsulated and represented by the term "Having-It-All", coined by Helen Gurley Brown, the first editor of Cosmopolitan magazine who published her book with the same title in 1982 (Gurley Brown 1982). The term, "Having-It-All" came to encompass the notion that women in contemporary society could aspire to have fulfilling, high-ranking careers and be mothers concurrently (Tropp 2006).

However, the term "Having It All" is experiencing a backlash from working women in the twenty-first century. There is a feeling that feminism is in need of reform and that "Having It All" is a misnomer. Women are aware that their gender and age affects the career choices they make and the opportunities that are offered to them, a fact that many contemporary feminists are addressing (e.g. Sandberg 2010). In an article in *The Atlantic* magazine titled "Why women still can't have it all", Ann-Marie Slaughter, the first female director of policy planning at the State Department wrote:

> "I was increasingly aware that the feminist beliefs on which I had built my entire career were shifting under my feet. ... when many members of the younger generation have stopped listening, on the grounds that glibly repeating "you can have it all" is simply airbrushing reality, it is time to talk". (Slaughter 2012)

It seems that as this first generation of career women have passed child-bearing age, many are sending a new message to the younger generation: think about the choices you are making while all the options are available to you. Indeed, in a survey undertaken for her book in 2002, Sylvia Hewlett found that in the USA 40% of women earning $50,000 or more a year are childless at age 45 (Hewlett 2004). Such a statistic would suggest that women have either chosen to be childless and have therefore focussed time and energy on furthering their career, or focussing on their career has distracted them from a previous desire to mother until it is "too late", a form of childless female identity Ireland refers to as "Transitional Women" (Ireland 1993: 41). Furthermore, such a statistic is highly suggestive that having a child severely limits women's chances of earning a high-level salary, which is in contrast to men who have children and women who do not, a fact that many women negotiating motherhood and career may be intuitively aware of.

In December 2014—the same year that Apple and Facebook announced that they would be offering egg freezing as an employee "benefit" to female employees in an effort to attract more women to their workforces—the New York Times reported that the percentage of American women in the workforce has been falling over the past decade and that 61 per cent of nonworking women cite family responsibilities as the reason (Cain Miller and Alderman 2014). Correspondingly, Carrie Lukas, a managing director of the Independent Women's Forum, wrote in her 2006 book about feminism: "*Feminist groups like to pretend that women can have it all without sacrificing time with families*" (Lukas 2006: 141), suggesting that Brown's book now looks like a charming artefact from a more hopeful time.

Scientific advances have enabled a shift in the way we approach motherhood (Tardy 2000). As a consequence, in recent years motherhood has become a choice available to us, when we choose it (Sevon 2005). In

October 2014 in an interview with the Telegraph, as Dr Geeta Nargund opened Europe's largest IVF clinic, she referred to fertility treatment as "the second wave of women's emancipation" (Peck 2014). As such, one possible way of viewing the current circumstance is as a "third wave" of feminism, one where motherhood is becoming one facet of female identity but not the whole story (Ireland 1993).

Exploring the Lived Experience

The Case of Sarah

Sarah is a 28-year-old woman working full time for a prominent digital news outlet.

Sarah is married and while determined to mother feels conflicted around the timing of motherhood at this stage in her life.

Sarah's experience of the phenomenon resonated with my own and in grappling with both of our telling it seemed there was a shared lived experience of anxiety overarching all aspects of the phenomenon. This experience of anxiety could be broadly divided into 3 themes: anxiety in the unknown, anxiety in meaning making and anxiety in temporality and finitude. Moreover, both of our experiences of anxiety could further be shown to exist on different levels of lived experience sitting in the 4 existential worlds (van Deurzen 2014).

This lived experience of anxiety, divided thematically, is depicted in the Table 12.1. Excerpts from the semi-structured conversation with Sarah have been inserted to illustrate the experience as it sits in the four worlds and in the three anxiety-related themes.

Uncertainty

A recurring theme expressed by Sarah around her lived experience of timing motherhood was a felt sense of uncertainty and unknowing. She portrayed a clear picture of her anxiety around the unknown nature of trying to plan and time motherhood while at the same time trying

Table 12.1 The experience of the anxiety of timing motherhood

	Anxiety "The paradox of freedom and finiteness"		
	Uncertainty	Meaning	Temporality/Finitude
Uberwelt *(Spiritual Dimension)*	"It is so unknown, my fertility - how long it will take".	"I feel like being a mother is what I'm here to do".	"Up until a certain age everything felt free and easy and then suddenly the seriousness and time pressure hits".
Mitwelt (Social Dimension)	"It never really struck me, I never thought about the logistics of things like ... mortgages and maternity leave - but now... what happens when we have a baby? Like, how do we afford the mortgage then?"	"I'd want to have a nice house, like I'm very traditional... I want to be married, owning a home, before we have a baby..."	"I've set myself this goal and I have to reach it before we start trying and... so I've basically put myself under immense amounts of pressure to get to this goal before September".
Eigenwelt (Personal Dimension)	"even though you have a husband or a partner... you're kind of on your own because it's your career, your desire, your passion and you have to decide, it's not up to anybody else..."	"caring for something entirely is the most important thing in the whole world, and I have this big desire to do that".	"I want to be where I know I'm going to stay with my career when I go on maternity, so I'm now in this kind of race to get out before we start trying..."

(continued)

Table 12.1 (continued)

	Anxiety "The paradox of freedom and finiteness"		
	Uncertainty	Meaning	Temporality/Finitude
Umwelt (Physical Dimension)	"And we've had conversations before where, she's said don't go into anything thinking about when you're going to have a baby because you haven't got a fucking clue where you're going to be" more, because I think, what if I can't do it, what if it doesn't happen for me…		"…he was putting together this book on fertility, and some of the stuff, I remember him coming home one day and saying I cannot believe how fast our eggs, well your eggs deteriorate… 35 there's a 70% chance that something will go wrong and how fast it goes to crap from 30 to 35, and so you kind of… don't want to be in the danger zone",

to make very definite decisions about her career progression. She also expressed the tension she experiences between her desire to plan and attempt to control the circumstances around becoming a mother and at the same time an awareness of the uncertainty of fertility and therefore timing conception.

In the following quote, Sarah shows her "worry" around her ability to conceive and her sense of not knowing when and if she will become a mother when she would like to:

> Yeh, you don't know how it's going to work… you've got no idea if it's going to work, and I don't think, I don't think a lot of people think… well I don't know if a lot of people think that way… um… but it is a big worry factor in my head, if I wasn't so worried about if I could, I don't know… because I am worried about if I could so that makes it more of a desire, because I want to do it and I want to make sure it gets done, it's like ticking a box…

She then continues to show how this uncertainty seems to impact the way she experiences other areas of her life, specifically career planning. A sense of anxiety is shown in the next quote as she explains how the uncertainty around when she will be able to conceive impacts how she feels about her ability to make decisions around her future career progression:

> Yeh… and that's really stressful, because that's like a… it's like constant… you can't just say, ok I'm going to quit my job on this day and go and do this [have a baby], it's not my choice… it's my choice to say ok lets start trying, but that's not to say that it's another 3 years down the line before we do anything, so then do you carry on looking for jobs in the time that you're trying? Do you sit pretty in the time that you're trying? Do you just get on with your life? Am I stuck at fucking **** [current employer] while I'm trying or what… you know, what the hell do I do?

Moreover, while Sarah has her own sense of anxiety in the uncertainty of timing motherhood, she also refers throughout our conversation to the impact of other women's experiences on her understanding of the uncertainty. In the quote below, she refers to a colleague who recently experienced a miscarriage and how watching her colleague's experience has in some way validated or supported her own sense of uncertainty and anxiety to make plans:

> And we've had conversations before where, she's [colleague] said don't go into anything thinking about when you're going to have a baby because you haven't got a fucking clue where you're going to be... um... and the same with houses, I was saying about houses and she was saying, well we thought we were going to have a baby in this house and we don't even know any more! So... that's kind of thrown it into turmoil in another way and it also makes me want it more, because I think, what if I can't do it, what if it doesn't happen for me...

Finitude and Temporality

The experience of anxiety in the uncertain nature of the phenomenon seems intrinsically linked to the inevitable finitude of fertility. For all women fertility has an end point, we are aware that there will come a time when conceiving and carrying a child will no longer be biologically viable. Yet, while we are aware that this time will come, exactly when it will be upon us is unknown and unknowable with any sureness. For this reason, there seems to be anxiety around a sense of time passing, the inevitability of this finitude and therefore an anxiety in the experience of ageing and temporality. In particular, age 30 has come to hold some significance for Sarah when conceptualising this anxiety. As such, Sarah references this age as a marker for her own positioning and understanding of where she is in her experience of the phenomenon. The extracts below show how Sarah conceptualises age 30 alongside the finitude of her fertility:

> Yeh... um... there is the fear, the ever growing fear that once you hit 30 your ovary's start to die, and everybody tells you this and everybody is screaming it and you get your mother who's from the baby boomers generation who's convinced of it, and is very much; you know you should really start thinking about it now.

> Yes… 30 is like, it really is like D-Day, it is like … that's it, whatever stage I'm at in career, whatever stage I'm at in my life, that is the deadline, and I have to start trying at that point, and if I'm not… I wanted to be pregnant at 30, and if I'm not at least trying… that's just not… that's not ever… it's just been my.. it's just been… 30.

Sarah shows how her age connects her to her own temporality. Age 30 seems to act as a marker and symbol in giving her a heightened sense of urgency in her decision around timing motherhood. In our conversation, Sarah explains how at this particular point in her life she feels as though all decisions need to be made quickly as there is a sense of time running out with the perceived deadline of age thirty hanging over her:

> Yeh… So it's like ok well I want to be at the pinnacle of my career or the place that I really want to be at… It's kind of like a goal, I've set myself this goal and I have to reach it before we start trying and… so I've basically put myself under immense amounts of pressure to get to this goal before September, even though September is probably not when we'll start trying anyway, so… but I'm 30 next June…

Throughout our conversation, Sarah expresses this felt sense of a deadline, and the resulting pressure she experiences as a result. Age thirty is conceptualised as a fertility marker, an age by which she feels her chances of conceiving a child will drop dramatically, and for this reason, the opportunity must be seized before the deadline. Moreover, Sarah's idea of the way in which childrearing and having a career interact and can coexist leads her to feel that her career must reach a "pinnacle" before she has a child. It seems that she believes this pinnacle must be reached in order to ensure the greatest possible career prospects following having a baby and maternity leave.

In terms of trying to "have-it-all", Sarah's experience seems to suggest that while she feels that she can try and juggle the roles of motherhood and work, she also has an underlying suspicion that to fulfil either to the best of her ability, one must suffer. This sentiment is expressed by Sarah and myself in the following extract:

> Um… And some of the best career women I've seen just don't have kids, they just don't do it…

Meaning

Sarah expressed a desire to mother that seems grounded in conceptualising motherhood as a life project that she feels is meaningful and essential. Sarah speaks about motherhood as a role that she believes would give her life ultimate purpose and is "*what [she] is here to do*". In our conversation, she explains her anxiety around the possibility of not becoming a mother due to either missing her opportunity as a result of career decisions or physically not being able. This feeling is demonstrated in the following extract:

> Whereas for me, it's like… I genuinely feel like it is what I'm here to do… And I love my career, I love my career, love my job, I love my life without a baby… But I feel like there is something in me that has to do it, I have to do it…

While this sentiment seems fairly straightforward, Sarah goes on to show how difficult and complex deciding how to live a life that feels meaningful is for her. She expresses the anxiety inherent in her grappling between a career and motherhood in terms of the fulfilment she believes each role will give her.

When Sarah expresses the importance she places on fulfilling the role of mother at the same time as feeling good about her career, I gained a clear understanding of her struggling with the questions and decisions around how she can live the most meaningful life. This grappling is shown in the following extract:

> and while I'm sure that changes once you've had a baby because you think oh I've got something more important in life, I don't want that, I want to have a career, I want to have something for me, and I've not spent my whole life working towards something to give up, like I will fight through this… um, and… and I don't know, I don't know how it's possible, I don't

> know how, I don't know anyone who has said they're going to be a certain way and stuck with it after having a baby...

This experience of anxiety in meaning making points to the notion of "having-it-all". The idea that women should be able to "have-it-all" has often implied that a combination of motherhood and career is the ultimate in meaningful female existence. I have been aware that my own experience of timing motherhood has been impacted by such a notion, with the underlying assumption being that to be *just* one or the other will not provide me with the ultimate experience of fulfilment that I seek, much like Sarah.

Conclusion

Anxiety is an inevitable part of the human condition. With this in mind, the lived experience of the anxiety in different situations must be illuminated and understood if we are to work well with clients and people experiencing them. With women's experiences notably neglected by much of the academic literature, a study such as this which explores and seeks to articulate an everyday female experience aims to enhance the work of practitioners working with young women.

Women around the age of 30 are increasingly presenting for psychotherapy and psychological support and therefore with a deeper understanding of the experiences they may be living through practitioners may be better equipped to support and make sense of the presenting issues.

References

Baird, D. T., Collins, J., Egozcue, J., Evers, L. H., Gianaroli, L., Leridon, H., et al. (2005). Fertility and Ageing. *Human Reproduction Update, 11*(3), 261–276. https://doi.org/10.1093/humupd/dmi006.

Boss, D. M., & Diethelm, O. (1949). *Meaning and Content of Sexual Perversions: A Daseinanalytic Approach to the Psychopathology of the Phenomenon of Love*. Trans. L. Lewis Abell. New York: Grune and Stratton. Retrieved from https://books.google.co.uk/books/about/Meaning_and_Content_of_Sexual_Perversion.html?id=QpXHXwAACAAJ&pgis=1.

Cain Miller, C., & Alderman, L. (2014, December 12). Why U.S. Women Are Leaving Jobs Behind. *The New York Times*.

Chodorow, N., & Contratto, S. (1992). The Fantasy of the Perfect Mother. In B. Thorne & M. Yalom (Eds.), *Rethinking the Family: Some Feminist Questions*. Boston, MA: Northeastern University Press.

Cohn, H. W. (2002). *Heidegger and the Roots of Existential Therapy*. London: Bloomsbury Academic.

de Beauvoir, S. (1949). *The Second Sex*. London: Random House.

Dillaway, H., & Parc, E. (2008). Locating Mothers: How Cultural Debates About Stay-at-Home Versus Working Mothers Define Women and Home. *Journal of Family Issues, 29*(4), 437–464. https://doi.org/10.1177/0192513X07310309.

Freud, S. (1905). *Three Essays on the Theory of Sexuality*. Se, 7.

Friedan, B. (2001). *The Feminine Mystique* (18th ed.). New York: W.W. Norton.

Greer, G. (1970). *The Female Eunuch*. London: HarperCollins.

Gurley Brown, H. (1982). *Having It All: Love, Success, Sex, Money Even If You're Starting with Nothing*. New York: Simon & Shuster.

Heidegger, M. (1927). *Being and Time*. Trans. J. Macquarrie & E. S. Robinson. London: Harper & Row.

Hewlett, S. A. (2004). *Creating a Life: What Every Woman Needs to Know About Having a Baby and a Career*. New York: Miramax Books. Retrieved from http://books.google.com/books?id=FFDyZDP-9mIC&pgis=1.

Ireland, M. S. (1993). *Reconceiving Women: Separating Motherhood from Female Identity*. New York: Guilford Press. Retrieved from http://books.google.com/books?id=UaeVxWNUoJYC&pgis=1.

Jackson, S. (2006). Interchanges: Gender, Sexuality and Heterosexuality—The Complexity (and Limits) of Heteronormativity. *Feminist Theory, 7*, 105–121.

Jacques, H. A., & Radtke, H. L. (2012). Constrained by Choice: Young Women Negotiate the Discourses of Marriage and Motherhood. *Feminism & Psychology, 22*(4), 443–461. https://doi.org/10.1177/0959353512442929.

Jaspers, K. (1951). *The Way to Wisdom*. New Haven, CT: Yale University Press.

Klay, M. A. (2009). Contemporary Women Turning 30. *Dissertation Abstracts Internations: Section B: The Sciences and Engineering*, *69*(10B), 6419.

Korula, G., & Mohan, S. K. (2010). Fertility and Age. *Journal of Human Reproductive Science, 3*(3), 121–123.

Langdridge, D., & Barker, M. (2013). Relationship Therapy with Lesbian, Gay, Bi and Trans Clients. In E. van Deurzen & S. Iacovou (Eds.), *Existential Perspectives on Relationship Therapy*. London: Routledge.

Lukas, C. (2006). *The Politically Incorrect Guide to Women, Sex, and Feminism.* Washington, DC: Regnery Publishing.

Macko, L., & Rubin, K. (2004). *Midlife Crisis at 30.* Emmaus, PA: Rodale Books.

Madankumar, R., Cohen, M. A., & Brenner, S. H. (2003). Age and Fertility. *Primary Care Update for OB/GYNS, 10*(6), 270–273. https://doi.org/10.1016/S1068-607X(03)00066-0.

Meyers, D. (2001). The Rush to Motherhood—Pronatalist Discourse and Women's Autonomy. *Signs: Journal of Women in Culture & Society*, *26* (3), 735–773.

Navot, D., & Bergh, P. A. (1991). Poor Oocyte Quality Rather than Implantation Failure as a Cause of Age Related Decline in Female Fertility. *Lancet, 337*(8754), 1375–1378.

Peck, S. (2014, October 27). Egg Freezing: The Perfect 30th Birthday Gift for Women. *The Telegraph*. Retrieved from http://www.telegraph.co.uk/women/womens-health/11188889/Egg-freezing-the-perfect-30th-birthday-gift-for-women.html.

Polt, R. (1999). *Heidegger: An Introduction.* Ithaca: Cornell University Press.

Raspberry, K. A., & Skinner, D. (2011 [1982]). Negotiating Desires and Options: How Mothers Who Carry the Fragile X Gene Experience Reproductive Decisions. *Social Science & Medicine*, *72*(6), 992–998. https://doi.org/10.1016/j.socscimed.2011.01.010.

Rich, A. (1986). *Of Woman Born.* New York, London: W.W. Norton.

Rich, A. C. (2003 [1980]). Compulsory Heterosexuality and Lesbian Existence. *Journal of Women's History*, *15*(3), 11–48. https://doi.org/10.1353/jowh.2003.0079.

Rowland, R. (1992). *Living Laboratories: Women and Reproductive Technology*. London: Cedar.

Sandberg, S. (2010). *Lean In: Women, Work, and the Will to Lead*. New York: Knopf Doubleday Publishing Group. Retrieved from http://books.google.co.uk/books/about/Lean_In.html?id=y9_mxZLYiiMC&pgis=1.

Segal, H. G., DeMeis, D. K., Wood, G. A., & Smith, H. L. (2001). Assessing Future Possible Selves by Gender and Socioeconomic Status Using the Anticipated Life History Measure. *Journal of Personality, 69*(1), 57–87. https://doi.org/10.1111/1467-6494.00136.

Sevon, E. (2005). Timing Motherhood: Experiencing and Narrating the Choice to Become a Mother. *Feminism & Psychology, 15*(4), 461–482. https://doi.org/10.1177/0959-353505057619.

Slaughter, A.-M. (2012). Why Women Still Can't Have It All. *The Atlantic*. Retrieved 23 July 2013, from http://www.theatlantic.com/magazine/archive/2012/07/why.

Tardy, R. W. (2000). "But I Am a Good Mom": The Social Construction of Motherhood through Health-Care Conversations. *Journal of Contemporary Ethnography, 29*(4), 433–473. https://doi.org/10.1177/089124100129023963.

Tone, A. (2001). *Devices & Desires: A History of Contraceptives in America*. New York: Hill and Wang.

Tropp, L. (2006). "Faking a Sonogram": Representations of Motherhood on Sex and the City. *The Journal of Popular Culture, 39*(5), 861–877. https://doi.org/10.1111/j.1540-5931.2006.00309.x.

van Deurzen, E. (2014). Structural Existential Analysis (SEA): A Phenomenological Research Method for Counselling Psychology. *Counselling Psychology Review, 29*(2), 70–83.

Warnock, M. (1970). *Existentialism*. Oxford: Oxford University Press.

Weixel-Dixon, K., & Strasser, F. (2005). Time and Purpose. In E. van Deurzen & C. Arnold-Baker (Eds.), *Existential Perspectives on Human Issues*. New York: Palgrave Macmillan.

Woollett, A., & Boyle, M. (2000). Reproduction, Women's Lives and Subjectivities. *Feminism & Psychology, 10*(3), 307–311. https://doi.org/10.1177/0959353500010003001.

Zornberg, A. G. (2009). *The Murmuring Deep: Reflections on the Biblical Unconscious (Google eBook)*. New York: Random House LLC. Retrieved from http://books.google.com/books?id=8UaQ4eyOFzEC&pgis=1.

13

The Experience of Being a Childfree Woman

Josephine Coates-Davies

Introduction

> There is very little agreement after all on what it is that constitutes, or ought to constitute, the category of women. (Butler 1990: 1)

In a book about the experiences of motherhood, it was deemed important to include a contrasting chapter, though immediately encountered is the problem of terminology. Language does not offer a satisfactory term for the women discussed here; child*less* points to a lack of something, child*free* has a sense of gleeful celebration that seems derogatory to mothers, *otherhood* cements the norm of motherhood, *non-mother* is merely stating what one isn't. Indeed, this latter point raises the question of why exploration of such a non-experience is necessary, or whether there is in fact a phenomenon to explore. This chapter is situated firmly within Part III of this book because it is the social and cultural impact

J. Coates-Davies (✉)
New School of Psychotherapy and Counselling, London, UK

C. Arnold-Baker (ed.), *The Existential Crisis of Motherhood*,
https://doi.org/10.1007/978-3-030-56499-5_13

of pronatalism that forces non-motherhood into a phenomenon in its own right. Despite the prevalence of research, media articles, books, Ted talks and blogs about this topic over the past thirty years, particularly by childfree women in frustrated response to assumptions made about them, it remains a phenomenon often met with criticism, judgement or bewilderment. It has also been shown that it is women, more than men, who meet with these societal responses, due to the way in which *woman* is seen to be synonymous with *mother*. Women who do not have children are not in themselves altogether unusual, but those who *deliberately* do not have children negate an array of assumptions that society holds about women whilst simultaneously existing within the structures that these assumptions have built. Being childfree (the less than satisfactory term I have opted for) therefore *becomes* a phenomenon by its very nature of being other to the norm of at least desiring motherhood if not achieving it. This chapter is based upon my phenomenological research into voluntarily as opposed to involuntarily childfree women due to the exploration of choice (Davies 2014). Although there is arguably a difference between the two groups, it will also be seen that the experience of being voluntarily childfree is not homogenous.

The Childfree Choice

There are many assumptions around the choice to be childfree, the first of which is that the word 'choice' is an accurate description of experience and another being that it is a simple binary choice between career and motherhood. Yet another is that it is a choice made by the individual woman alone. All of these are erroneous. The experience of becoming childfree is multifaceted, socially situated and unique to each individual. To begin with, I will deconstruct the notion of 'choice'.

Paradoxically, it is the women who feel most certain that they don't and will never want children whose childfree position in the world is most commonly described as childfree by *choice*. But it is precisely the strength of conviction about not wanting children that puts the word *choice* in doubt; it is more of an automatic, or *default* position that is unchanging and doesn't seem open to the option of motherhood. It is a non-thing that holds far more significance for others than for the individual. Thus, 'choice' isn't a particularly good description for this experience as the term denotes a decision-making process wherein two or more options are available and there is a need or desire to select between them. For these women there is only surety, there is no decision-making; childfreedom is felt to be a foregone conclusion because without the desire or intent to mother, childfreedom is merely a consequence of their being who they are, and *motherhood* would be the experienced choice. However, due to the aforementioned societal presumption of woman being synonymous with mother, those who are not mothers are often required to account for themselves. Indeed, the belief in all women having an automatic desire for children is so deeply embedded in the collective psyche that it can lead the unambivalent women into doubt about the validity of their absence of desire, perhaps even questioning whether this indicates deficiency or lack of femininity.

Secondly are the women who have no particularly strong feelings one way or the other—children are not considered to be essential to life, and motherhood doesn't *matter* to them. Instead, other aspects of life matter deeply, such as seeking meaning through activities unrelated to the traditional paths of marriage and family, or developing a stable relationship in which children might or might not then be had (Davies 2014). This means that choices are made in life that might *result* in being childfree, but childfreedom itself does not feel like the thing that has been chosen per se. Although these women are often described as ambivalent, in fact the opposite is true; ambivalence derives from the Latin roots of two words—*ambi* meaning both, and *valence* meaning strong—it is to be pulled in two opposing directions or 'on the horns of a dilemma'. But these women are not pulled in any particular direction with regard to this phenomenon so perhaps a more fitting term would be *neque-valent* from the Latin words 'neither' and 'strong'; neither of these life choices are felt to be of great concern and these women are unsure as to where they fit on the spectrum of choice (ibid.)

Finally, there are the women for whom the choice is deeply existential—those who are truly ambivalent in the literal translation of the word. The mutually exclusive paths of motherhood and non-motherhood hold equal value, each option is different, but not of more or less value than the other. *Choice* now becomes a profoundly apt term, a necessary process affecting the person's whole being in which "the colourful palette of motivation may emerge only in a canvas of black or white" (Davies 2014: 97). The individual may oscillate between the opposing poles and this can be exhausting and frustrating. For some there is an active wish for passivity—for the decision to somehow be taken out of her hands such as the fantasy of finding a baby in a basket on the doorstep (Davies 2014). However, despite the wish for passivity, the choice between motherhood and being childfree still matters, therefore the ownership of the choice is greatly important despite the struggle involved. For example, in relationships there is a need to negotiate a continuing freedom to choose rather than have the option shut down by a partner's choice. This is an interesting paradox that highlights the nature of human beings as process rather than essence; there is extension of the person, and unfolding of the self, from the situation of the present into the possibility of the future (Heidegger 1927). For the women in the preceding paragraphs, this is not an aspect of self that matters; thus, there is no need to engage in the process of choice, of becoming rather than being childfree. But for the women currently discussed, there is a difference between an ongoing process, which may transiently be experienced as a need for passivity, versus the end of process—the reification or cementing of this aspect of the self. It is having the option of what Sartre (1943) describes as 'choosing not to choose' as opposed to having the choice taken away entirely. In choosing not to choose the person may be acting within an 'inauthentic' mode of being (Heidegger 1927), but this is against the backdrop of an 'authentic' mode in which there remains ownership of choice. Therefore, though there are times when having the choice taken away feels seductive, this feeling is not exclusive; there are also times when being in the authentic mode requires an engagement with the ongoing process of choice despite the difficulty this entails.

Maternal Instinct

The idea of the person as process as opposed to essence is interesting in that it contradicts a deeply rooted cultural belief which is often referred to as 'maternal instinct' or 'biological imperative', and which places *all* women in the position of mothers-to-be in terms of their desire and potential. It is a way of 'essentialising', or predetermining the female pathway through life and contributes to the sense of stigma around the *choice* to be childfree as this negates the belief in a fundamental essence of being female. Sartre's description of the person illuminates this particular tension; he describes human existence as *pour-soi* (for-itself), meaning a being conscious of itself, as lacking essence and therefore incomplete. This lack of essentiality, or 'nothingness' at the heart of being, gives rise to existential anxiety that we strive to eliminate by reducing ourselves to *en-soi* (in-itself), a complete thing that no longer has the freedom to choose and the anxiety that necessitates (Sartre 1943). Notions of an instinct or biological drive fall into an essentialist perspective, and though it may well have phenomenological applicability to the experience of *some* women, it is by no means universal, negating the usefulness or accuracy of the term itself. Thus whilst the belief in maternal instinct often creates a social tension for those who do not experience this urge, it may also serve as an avoidance of existential tension for others who hold a more essentialist view. It is perhaps easier to label with pathology, to pity or to scorn women whose childfree choice is based upon absence of desire to mother, than to recognise that *naturalness* does not necessarily have to dictate one's choices.

The notion of the nurturing, maternal mother figure is so pervasive that it can either position childfree women as other to the norm through a process of making them deficient, lacking something that other, 'normal' women experience, or attempts to include them in a way that makes their choices more palatable but denies the autonomy of the individual. For example, a childfree woman's relationships with children may be perceived as being a way of satisfying her innate need to nurture that has been thwarted in the absence of motherhood. This encapsulates the essentialist view of women's lives as dictated by a feminine nature, but ignores the phenomenology of what *does* exist for the individual; it is a way of fitting otherness into the traditional definition of 'woman' without needing to extend the definition itself.

'Maternal instinct' is also existentially problematic as it proffers a duality between self and body, with specific applicability to the female sex, denying female agency by presupposing a one-dimensional urge that overwrites other facets of choice. As Simone de Beauvoir (1949) describes, the female experience is regarded as that of 'immanence', as wholly immersed in the inner world of the body as opposed to the male experience which is transcendent of the body and focused upon the external world. Thus inner and outer, immanence and transcendence, become female and male polarities and biology is seen to be the defining factor of being female, the heart of which is being-towards-motherhood. In reality however, women and men alike are beyond this immanent-transcendent duality; each is individually impacted by their subjective and objective experiences and there is no such thing as a person, including the female and her biology, as separate from the world.

But herein lies a curious paradox; though women are viewed in this way as wholly subjective beings, historically *man* is subject against which woman is other, or object (de Beauvoir 1949). This is a peculiar tension of the intersection between the personal and the social dimensions and affects facets of life including identity, sexuality and ideals of femininity. The common factor in this apparent contradiction is that of woman as *being-for-others;* seen as the naturally nurturing mother figure she primarily serves her children; and seen as the object of sexuality she is primarily for the eyes of the (male) gaze (ibid.). Therefore, serving others assumes the position of a natural trait of femininity, leading to an automatic polarisation of 'selfishness' in those who choose to forego mothering and all its attendant duties.

Ethics

This idea of selfishness may also become synonymous with hedonism, or the assumption of a life of individualised luxury. For example, the August 2013 cover of *Time Magazine* featured an attractive young couple lying on the beach under the caption *The Childfree Life: when having it all means not having children* (Sandler 2013). This provoked a strong response, particularly from religious speakers but matching a more general trend, against a life that places freedom above values, and arguing that each individual should transcend their 'private desire' for freedom from the duty of parenthood in order to contribute to the wider of context of community and God (Fr. Barron 2013; Kirchgaessner 2015). In fact, both perspectives hold assumptions—either about the notion of private desire or the polarity of freedom and value—that do not match the experience of childfree women and can be critiqued from an existential standpoint.

Private Desire

The perspective of the childfree choice as selfish or immature is ingrained in different parts of culture—religiously, as Fr. Barron outlines, it is our duty to serve God and the community. In addition, many early developmental theories place parenthood, particularly motherhood, as the pinnacle of personal development, and the absence of desire for a child as indicative of pathology (Freud 1924; Jung 1938; Erikson 1950). Indeed, these perceptions are often adopted by childfree women themselves as they acknowledge the unappealing aspects of parenthood they are grateful to avoid, such as not being tied down in life. The pervasive polarisation of being either nurturing or selfish means that the absence of the selflessness of parenthood indicates the presence of the selfishness of non-parenthood. But upon deeper analysis it is discovered that it is only one part of the word's meaning—putting oneself first—that is relevant. The second part—*lacking consideration for other people*—is rejected as being entirely inappropriate as many childfree women strongly state that it would be deeply unethical to have children *before* one is ready, or within an unstable relationship, or with a partner who may be immature him or herself, or within a catastrophically overpopulated earth (Davies 2014). Furthermore, psychoanalytic and developmental theories that isolate the individual from the world by placing 'motherhood' as an abstract pinnacle to be attained do not fit the lived experience of women's decision-making which revolve around the concrete reality of a child, even an as yet hypothetical one, as a person whose well-being is of primary importance and thus at the very heart of choice. It may be stated therefore, that the choice to be childfree is often not based solely upon the individual's private desire, but is fundamentally rooted in the social world. Once again, a 'natural' position is assumed but not analysed—parenthood, like heterosexuality, is the 'base' against which alternatives are situated, but the base itself escapes the same deconstruction because of its assumed naturalness.

Freedom and Values

However, when childfreedom *does* stem from a more subjective stance, freedom might be something stated as either a motivation for being childfree or as an unexpected and appreciated result. But there is a difference here between the more generic, culturally understood sense of freedom that is carefree or responsibility free, and the existential sense of having freedom within the limitations of existence, including anxious acknowledgement of our time-bound existence for which we are responsible for creating ourselves in action. Part of this existential responsibility is to question the meaning of one's own life, and consider how best to live within or without societal constraints. Meaning may or may not be found in parenting, and both motherhood and childfreedom hold the potential for authentic or inauthentic engagement with responsibility and authenticity, and it is *this* process, rather than the need for literal freedom, that many childfree women speak of. Although there is sometimes acknowledgement that motherhood would be deeply meaningful, it is not the primary place that meaning is sought and though this search for meaning *does* stem from a subjective stance, or *inwardness* (Kierkegaard 1843), it is also borne out of an authenticity that encourages the individual towards commitment to her own values in areas other than motherhood. Having children, though conforming to a social norm, would not be the authentically subjective route, based as it would be on the preferences or injunctions of others rather than stemming from the individual's own values.

The Road Not Travelled

The assumed centrality of motherhood to women's lives gives rise to another pervasive discourse—the inevitability of regret—which again conflicts with the lived experience of childfree women. The term 'regret' has a threefold definition of sadness, repentance and disappointment (OED 2018) and emphasises the *authorship* of the action or non-action that is regretted. Interestingly, the definition of *existential* regret opposes this in its emphasis on the *non-authorship* of that which is regretted. Lucas (2004) defines the latter term as the negative feelings around past choices that are seen as inauthentic or as failing to follow one's value system, or indeed the non-choices borne out of a need to choose not to choose (Sartre 1943). This latter point elucidates the kind of futile circularity childfree women have when questioning whether or not they might regret their choice in the future; the past or present choice is in accordance with the values and authentic position of the individual thus cannot be subject to *existential* regret in the future, and the former definition seems to be too abstract as it requires an imagined change of authentic position. Of course, this is not to say there aren't those who *do* regret being childfree, but the possibility of regret is another of life's unavoidable existential tensions due to the need to make choices in the absence of knowledge about the outcome of those choices. As Kierkegaard puts it; "It is quite true what philosophy says: that life must be understood backwards. But then one forgets the other principle: that it must be lived forwards" (Kierkegaard 1843: 161). In this instance, it is society that warns of the need to understand backwards from the perspective of the future, but it is the forwardness in the present which must also be taken into account in order to live according to one's current values.

However, the inapplicability of the term 'regret' does not mean that feelings are altogether excluded. For some childfree women there is a sense of loss in what was not chosen, curiosity about the experience of motherhood, or an acknowledgement that a life in which there is a struggle to create meaning could have felt differently with the addition of children and grandchildren (Davies 2014). But these questions and feelings do not equate to the term 'regret' as defined above. Instead, there is an engagement with the existential truth of choice equating to sacrifice, and recognition that not every path can be travelled; it is an ineluctable aspect of the human condition that "'Things fade' and 'Alternatives exclude'" (Gardner 1971: 133). Indeed, there is a sense that these feelings, or 'longings' enrich our lives, guide us towards further seeking of fulfilment and authorship of our lives—it is the power of authentic choice (McLeod 2017). Before moving on from this section, it is interesting to briefly note the far greater emphasis upon and anxiety around the possible regret for being childfree over that of becoming a mother; though there are most certainly those who do regret having children, and this remains one of society's strongest taboos (Hager 2011; Donath 2015).

Legacy

Gardner's aforementioned, remarkably existential phrase is preceded by another; "The ultimate evil is that Time is perpetual perishing, and being actual involves elimination" (Gardner 1971: 132). Though applicable to all living things, humans are the only beings who have awareness of this aspect of being, thus it becomes a defining component of our psyche and a concern for how we live our lives and how we die our deaths. Yalom (1980) argues that we spend a great deal of time attempting to avoid the knowledge of our certain demise through illusionary tactics such as a belief in our specialness or in an ultimate rescuer, and that this may also lead to an ongoing concern with leaving a legacy, or a part of us that lives on after our death. Paradoxically, although it is women who experience the most warnings of regret, it is *men* who are understood to have the strongest need to pass on their genetic legacy. This could merely be a reflection of patriarchal conditioning, wherein the male experience has traditionally been given primacy over the female (Johnson 2014), but it is also important to consider the meaning of legacy through an existential lens.

In discussing our relationships with the past, van Deurzen observes how contemporary individualist societies have become increasingly unknowledgeable and potentially uncaring about lineage and ancestry, and how this lack of knowledge of the past may impact upon our ability to imagine the future; "our roots these days are shorter, our vision tends to follow" (van Deurzen-Smith 1997: 115). This is echoed in a more recent article by writer Lionel Shriver who argues that it is the cultures in which the childfree choice is predominantly made, white Westerners, that heritage is taken for granted and we have become 'a-historical' (Shriver 2015). These cultures are ageing as the birth rate declines whilst the average age of death increases, adding to the sense that the childfree choice is a selfish one.

Meaning

However, although some childfree women, particularly those without siblings, question the significance of being the end of their genetic line, it often remains an intellectual question rather than an emotional one—they are generally unmoved by the idea of legacy (Davies 2014). The participants in my own research did not equate the lack of meaning they found in the idea of legacy with a wider sense of meaninglessness per se, but this is not always the case. In one of the few chapters on this topic by a male writer, tellingly entitled *The End of the Line*, Tim Kreider posits that to refrain to have children is one of the most illogical decisions a person can make because it instantly renders life meaningless (Kreider 2015). He echoes Yalom's description of the human temptation towards hiding from our own mortality, adding that although reproduction is the main purpose of any living species, for humans it has the added benefit of being a particularly good way of maintaining the illusion of immortality through the continuation of one's genes and therefore somehow also oneself. Thus, to remain childfree is to "constitute a kind of existential vanguard, forced by our own choices to face the naked question of existence with fewer illusions, or at least fewer consolations, than the rest of humanity" (Kreider 2015: 274). Returning to Heidegger's work however, it is clear that each of us as individuals must engage and disengage with the knowledge of our mortality in a constant oscillation between authenticity and inauthenticity (Heidegger 1927). Additionally, we must each create meaning through our own ventures, and though it may be true that many parents find meaning in their children, they are not necessarily more immune to the existential tensions of life than non-parents.

Temporality

The above discussion is one in which I have avoided posing a difference between the sexes because they each are subject to the human condition of temporality. But female biology is again assumed to mean a fundamental difference in that the menopause will trigger strong feelings for childfree women regarding the end of the potential to become a biological mother (Trethewey 2001). However, the biological end of possibility is firstly not a homogenous experience, and secondly does not necessarily coincide with the feeling of ending. Research shows that some women, despite having never wanted children, experience a feeling of a door closing, and a finality that shifts their sense of identity from the process of 'not having children' to the cementation of '*did not have children*' (Morell 1994; Delyser 2007). Conversely, my own research found that the choice to be childfree was with a single exception felt to be finalised within the thirties. By age forty, regardless of ongoing biological potential to become pregnant, the women had already defined themselves as permanently childfree, and for those who had struggled with the choice, entering the forties was felt as a relief, and a lifting of the burden of choice (Davies 2014).

It is of course true that there are biological, social and cognitive elements to this earlier decision-making in people's acknowledgement of declining fertility rates into the forties, as well as the social and cognitive elements of clocking one's own age against the imagined future of ongoing parenting. Nonetheless, there is an additional, existential element to consider, which is most easily done by turning to the work of Martin Heidegger, a philosopher whose description of the person is largely genderless and ageless, but who dedicated a vast portion of his thinking to the notion of temporality, or human experience of time. For Heidegger (1927), time is the phenomenon against which *all* human experience must be considered, and fundamentally, time is not linear in terms of past preceding present followed by future. Instead, there is a unity of the three dimensions of time such that the present includes knowledge of and projection into the future as well as a relationship with the past. In this way, the person is not confined to the present, regardless of what biological or social experiences it encompasses. Instead, the person exists in what Heidegger terms 'primordial' time. It is one's *ownmost* temporality, the finite rather than eternal sense (and sensing) of time that ends with one's own death. Heidegger binds together these ideas by stating "Time must be brought to light – and genuinely conceived – as the horizon for all understanding of Being and for any way of interpreting it" (Heidegger 1962: 39).

To separate biology from the whole sphere of one's existence is to diminish the meaning and existential understanding that the individual has of her life in its totality. And yet to discount the knowledge women have of their finite fertility is also to diminish their existential reality. Again, there are overlapping threads of life that cannot be pulled free of the entire tapestry without rendering it nonsensical.

Sociality

The final part to consider here, the social aspect of being childfree, has been a continuous strand throughout the discussion so far, given that the personal and social cannot be viewed discretely, but there is one further element to discuss in terms of a tension between the two realms.

van Deurzen-Smith (1997) outlines two fundamental aspects of the social world as belonging and acceptance, the poles of which are isolation and rejection. It is unsurprising therefore that the identity of being childfree by *choice*, with the attendant potential for stigma, may be disowned in favour of the less risky identity of childfree by circumstance. Park (2002) described this as 'passing', wherein one's choices are not voiced and the assumptions made by others, namely fertility problems, are allowed. However, van Deurzen follows on to describe two fundamental aspects of the *personal* world as being integrity and identity, which may be negatively impacted upon by the choice to avoid rejection by others. One's integrity may be deeply entwined with one's sense of authenticity, including ownership of the choice to be childfree, and that to pass oneself off as infertile or circumstantially childless is to conceal an important aspect of identity. Thus, a tension arises and a secondary ongoing choice is needed—how to navigate the social world in terms of ownership or non-ownership of choice, and the degree to which one is comfortable with risking rejection or criticism for that choice. This is further complicated by the myriad ways in which women become childfree, where they feel they are situated on the spectrum of choice, and how they experience themselves in this regard.

Conclusion

The experience of becoming and being childfree is the point at which the personal and social worlds meet and which cannot be said to be homogenous with regard to any of the existentials of life, including meaning and meaninglessness, freedom and choice, responsibility, authenticity, temporality or sociality. It is celebrated, condemned, important and unimportant. It is chosen with deeply difficult consideration and absolute ease. It is a phenomenon harmful to certain ageing cultures and essential to an overpopulated planet. It is perhaps a current fascination that will lessen in terms of its impact as diversity becomes the norm in more social spheres. It is perhaps an inevitable result of the existential age—an age in which we no longer have the certainty of God and a belief in eternal reward for a life of toil, where in the individualistic cultures of the West we elevate the individual over the group, and celebrate progression towards the future whilst simultaneously attempt to maintain our rootedness in the past. Childfreedom is therefore also a tension, an existential standpoint that is impossible to ignore, that invites questioning yet is deeply personal, that is an individual's choice yet impacts the choices of others, that negates the synonymity of woman and mother and demonstrates that women are not exempt from the notion of contextual being, are not necessarily more *essence* than men. Perhaps the truest conclusion is that if we allow ourselves as a society to look beyond tradition and essentialism, we may realise that the differences between us are far less important than the similarities, and that the choice to be or not to be a mother does not necessitate a barrier to understanding each other.

References

Barron, Fr. R. (2013). *The Very Sad Childfree Life*. [Online]. Real Clear Religion. Available at http://www.realclearreligion.org/articles/2013/09/09/the_very_sad_childfree_life.html (Accessed 4 May 2014).

Butler, J. (1990 [2006]). *Gender Trouble* (2nd ed.). New York: Routledge.

Davies, J. (2014). *A Phenomenological Exploration into the Lived Experience of Childfree Women Aged 45–55*. Doctorate in Existential Psychotherapy, Middlesex University, London.

De Beauvoir, S. (1949 [2009]). *The Second Sex*. Trans. from French by C. Borde & S. Malovany-Chevallier. London: Random House.

Delyser, G. (2007). *Experiences at Midlife of Intentionally Childfree Women*. Ph.D. Institute for Clinical Social Work, Chicago, IL.

Donath, O. (2015). Regretting Motherhood: A Sociopolitical Analysis. *Signs Journal of Women in Culture and Society, 40*(2), 343–367.

Erikson, E. (1950 [1963]). *Childhood and Society* (2nd ed.). New York: W. W. Norton.

Freud, S. (1924 [1991]). The Dissolution of the Oedipus Complex. In *On Sexuality: Three Essays on the Theory of Sexuality and Other Works*. Trans. from German by J. Stachey. London: Penguin Books.

Gardner, J. (1971 [1989]). *Grendel*. London: Vintage Books.

Hager, T. (2011). Making Sense of an Untold Story: A Personal Deconstruction of the Myth of Motherhood. *Qualitative Inquiry, 17*(6), 35–44.

Heidegger, M. (1927 [1962]). *Being and Time*. Trans. from German by J. Macquarrie & E. S. Robinson. London: Harper and Row.

Johnson, A. G. (2014). *The Gender Knot: Unravelling Our Patriarchal Legacy*. Pennsylvania: Temple University Press.

Jung, C. G. (1938). *Four Archetypes*. Trans. from German by R. F. C. Hull. London: Routledge.

Kierkegaard, S. (1843 [1992]). *Either/Or: A Fragment of Life*. Trans. from Danish by A. Hannay. London: Penguin Books.

Kierkegaard, S. (1843). *Papers and Journals*. Trans. from Danish by A. Hannay (43 IV A 164).

Kirchgaessner, S. (2015, February). Pope Francis: Not Having Children Is Selfish. *The Guardian* [online]. Available at https://www.theguardian.com/world/2015/feb/11/pope-francis-the-choice-to-not-have-children-is-selfish (Accessed 9 December 2018).

Kreider, T. (2015). The End of the Line. In M. Daum (Ed.), *Selfish, Shallow, and Self-Absorbed; Sixteen Writers on the Decision Not to Have Kids*. New York: Picador.

Lucas, M. (2004). Existential Regret: A Crossroads of Existential Anxiety and Existential Guilt. *Journal of Humanistic Psychology, 44*(1), 58–70.

McLeod, V. (2017). *Childless by Choice: A Powerful Act of Fulfilment*. Ted Talk [Video online]. Available at https://www.youtube.com/watch?v=TKOKD69jUA0 (Accessed 10 August 2018).

Morell, C. M. (1994). *Unwomanly Conduct: The Challenges of Intentional Childlessness*. London: Routledge.

OED Online. Oxford University Press. (2018, December). Available at https://en.oxforddictionaries.com/definition/regret (Accessed 9 December 2018).

Park, K. (2002). Stigma Management Among the Voluntarily Childless. *Sociological Perspectives., 45*(1), 21–45.

Sandler, L. (2013, August). The Childfree Life: When Having It All Means Not Having Children. *Time Magazine* 182(7).

Sartre, J. P. (1943 [1969]). *Being and Nothingness: An Essay on Phenomenological Ontology.* Trans. from French by H. E. Barnes. London: Routledge.

Shriver, L. (2015). Be Here Now Means Be Gone Later. In M. Daum (Ed.), *Selfish, Shallow, and Self-Absorbed; Sixteen Writers on the Decision Not to Have Kids*. New York: Picador.

Trethewey, A. (2001). Reproducing and Resisting the Master Narrative of Decline: Midlife Professional Women's Experiences of Aging. *Management Communication Quarterly, 15*(2), 183–226.

van Deurzen-Smith, E. (1997). *Everyday Mysteries: Existential Dimensions of Psychotherapy*. London: Routledge.

Yalom, I. D. (1980). *Existential Psychotherapy*. New York: Basic Books.

Part IV

Working with Existential Crisis in Clinical Practice

14

Exploring the Moods of First Time Mothers Through Imagery

Aoife Gaffney

Introduction

From the moment we are born, we are 'thrown' into the world of emotional experiences (Heidegger 1962). Emotions are both an intimate and intimidating phenomenon that can influence our choices and actions. Valued above all, at least within contemporary neoliberal society, are positive emotions, yet existentialists do not valorise certain emotions over others. Instead, all feelings and emotions are considered relevant in creating lived experiences, which are always in flux. At the same time, existential theory does not discount an individual's difficulties, or in this case, a mother's struggles. It does not minimise a person, so can easily recognise without judgment that mothers experience difficult and unpleasant emotions. Existential theory contends that these emotional experiences have their place and that even the most challenging moods can reveal us to ourselves (Fig. 14.1).

A. Gaffney (✉)
Psychology Department, Dublin Business School, Dublin, Ireland

C. Arnold-Baker (ed.), *The Existential Crisis of Motherhood*,
https://doi.org/10.1007/978-3-030-56499-5_14

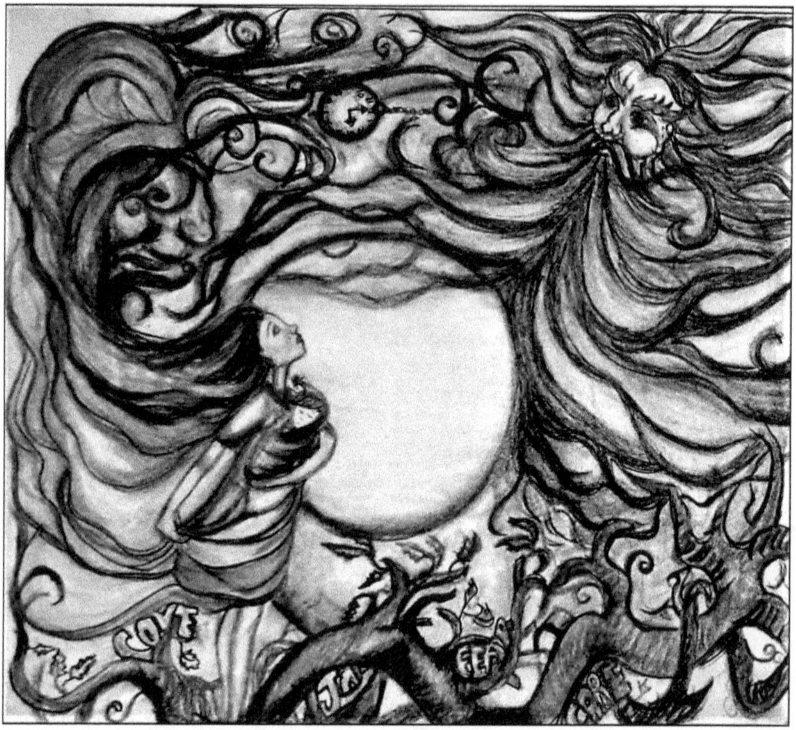

Fig. 14.1 The Windy Weather of Motherhood (Gaffney 2019)

My research focused on eight first-time mothers living in Ireland and their experiences of mood and emotion—as revealed through images. Creative methods offer a unique model for exploring the lived experience of emotion and mood, enriching the understanding of the phenomenon from an existential perspective. Clinically, Existential Psychology and Art Therapy practices possess many similarities. Both are interested in opening up the client's possibilities and worldviews. They recognise the uniqueness of each person, and therefore, defy reductive ways of viewing lived experience and in this case, a mother's experience of motherhood.

This chapter considers how first-time mothers experience mood and emotion as well as how therapists can work with postnatal difficulties in clinical practice from an existential creative position. The chapter introduces the concept of mood briefly before discussing two themes from my research study. A concluding section briefly explores ways of working with mood and motherhood from a creative existential perspective.

The Mood of Motherhood

Motherhood is challenging and is a significant life transition that requires extensive personal, physical, social and spiritual modification and rectification. These profound changes, of course, occasion emotional fluctuations. Emotion, as Deurzen explains, is a 'good place to start to understand a person's worldview' (van Deurzen 2009: 141). Moods are the weather of the world, sweeping through in changeable fronts of storms or sunshine. 'Extreme' weather events, of course, draw the most attention (van Deurzen 2009: 141), and like mood can threaten to swell and create an unpleasant atmosphere, which in its extreme form cause harm or damage.

Nevertheless, 'rather than dividing emotions into good and bad ones and aiming for the good ones' Deurzen argues, 'we need to learn to get the hang of each position on our emotional compass so that we can guide ourselves through the complexity of life' (ibid.). Emotions in motherhood, especially negative ones, are generally linked to psychopathology or mental health difficulties. Most of the research on emotions and moods in motherhood has focused on the medical discourses surrounding such postpartum disorders as postnatal depression and postnatal anxiety. From an existential perspective, extreme or fluctuating emotion in the face of real or imaginary danger is one of the most fundamental human experiences (ibid.: 98). Nevertheless, at present, postpartum research does not consider the idea that emotion is energy, an emblem of being alive, nor that angst and dread might be desirable as a source of energy (ibid.). Facing the depth of existence can offer a new vantage point on the truth in life (ibid.). Thus, from an existential vantage point, it is possible to fall to rock bottom, to rise again. Loss, according to Kierkegaard (1844), can propel someone forward in search of their values. As Kierkegaard famously wrote, anxiety is the 'dizziness of freedom' (Kierkegaard 1844: 75) which ultimately helps us realise our possibilities. Depression, in contrast, arises from the erosion of freedom—a familiar story for some mothers. One's time is not one's own, and decisions are always made with the baby in mind. What a mother wears, when she can sleep, eat or shower is always in pre-contemplation and conditional upon the needs of another.

Consequently, becoming a mother may strip bare the truth, revealing the reality of responsibility. One's existence becomes illuminated. This is not necessarily negative, but rather a recognition of how the world works. Embracing existential feelings offers an alternative perspective on the subject of mood that does not pathologise fear, dread, sadness, loss, or other supposedly 'negative' feelings. Thus, neither state—angst or depression—needs to be pathologised, but instead may be recognised as essential to a new and richer understanding of existence. Motherhood is a heart-warming, beautiful and fulfilling experience in part because it can produce the anxiety of living. A mother can recognise and affirm her new state of *Being:* I am anxious. I am a mother. I am alive. Thus, to be a person and to be a mother is to recognise possibility and necessity then move between the two. The everyday state for a mother is to be in a mood, and it is not extraordinary to feel intense emotion. In fact, it is ordinary.

Research Findings

As part of my research, I interviewed eight first-time mothers individually, to gain an understanding into the experience of mood and emotion. The research was also invested in using a creative data collection method (drawing/painting), which was complementary to the interpretative phenomenological framework. The interview process was completed in stages. At our first meeting, the women were given the same instruction regarding the creation of an image: 'create an image of your personal experience of motherhood and while creating the image, think of your mood and emotions'. I deliberately used the word 'image' to signal that the research was not about creative or artistic ability, a point I also verbally emphasised to co-researchers. All of the mothers (Rebecca,

Daisy, Danielle, Lucy, Sarah, Grace, Maggie and Hannah) completed an image (drawing/painting) prior to the semi-structured interviews, which were conducted on an individual basis (approximately a month later). The participating mother was then invited to discuss her image. Each interview then opened with the following question: 'Can you tell me about the image that you created in as much detail as possible?' Subsequent questions were flexibly posed in response to what the co-researchers stated. Questions about the co-researcher's emotions and mood were often asked for clarification. For example, when a co-researcher was exploring an event, a follow-up question would often explore how she felt. Images were analysed as single cases initially and then compared. I found that the images opened-up a unique reflective space for the mothers, and through the image and narratives, I discovered that their individual maternal realities contained many layers of emotional experience and representation.

Consequently, a broad, flexible and innovative structure of image analysis was employed to interpret the mother's worldview as depicted in the image (see Table 14.2). The approach was inspired by Deurzen and Adams theory of existential dreamwork (2011), which maintains that truth derives from the meaning attributed by the creator in the first instance, and not (in this case) the researcher. To realise this, an Interpretative Phenomenological Analysis (IPA) methodology was utilised as the principal framework. The women's images are briefly described next, with particular focus on the elements that are representative of the two themes—the 'mammy worry' and the 'existential shift of emotions'.

Visual Depictions

The 'mammy worry' pervades the co-researchers' images yet takes different forms. Rebecca portrays her worry as a monster-like figure: 'the worry monster'. She also depicts what she calls the vortex, a swirl of darkness with bright yellow circles within it. The vortex contains the darkness and holds the 'brighter' parts of her emotional experience. In contrast, a balance is struck within the image and on the right-hand side of the page a serene image of nature, representing the day when it all goes to plan.

Daisy's worry is expressed through the words written on her picture, 'fear', 'expectations' 'uncertainty', 'frustration', 'love', 'hope', 'joy' and 'responsibility'. The leading figure in the image is 'Winnie the Pooh'. He is holding three brightly coloured balloons, and as he flies through the air he is supported by a pair of hands, which are faintly drawn. While the 'holding hands' in her image represents her supporting and protecting, they also carry the weight of responsibility.

For Danielle, the crippling darkness of the cave on the right-hand side of the page, the naked, wounded figure, stabbed in the back and crying a river of blood. In the prone position, she is vulnerable and alone except for the dark butterfly tethered to the cave, which evokes the gnawing uncertainty of the unknown. This is in contrast to the serenity of the dyad of mother and baby and the brightly coloured surround, which represents times of playfulness and fun.

For Lucy, the image is of a window representing her thoughts and feelings. The window is further divided into four panes of glass, and each pane contains a different image. The images portrayed are, a broken-cracked heart, teardrops, clasped hands, a pair of lips and a pair of eyes with 'zzz' hovering above them. There are also questions being asked, with question marks depicted floating in space. Each of the question marks and teardrops within the image depicts both her worry and her expression of it.

Sarah like Lucy also divides her page. The central figure has a big smile, but in contrast, there is a black cloud, which looms beside her. Her depiction of a heart is vivid and red but again surrounded by a dark circle. Tears, rainbows and flowers make up the bottom section and add vibrancy to her image. This is marked still by the dark symbols, again representing the bright and the darker emotions.

For Grace, the need to be grounded in her image is presented by the floor of pebbles, and the natural world, which represent her roots and her family. Her image is of plants alive and growing, but with some coloured brown rather than green. Most of the objects are known to her, but there is one that she is unsure of; a protruding plant reaching in towards the organic representation of mother and babe. Time passing is represented by yellow pods (circles), which are shrouded in shading—drifting into the distance.

Maggie draws her worry as waves. The black squiggles and smoke-like lines rise from the bed placed in the centre of the page. A balancing scale tips in the corner. Her lack of sleep is evident in the image and illuminates her everyday struggle.

Finally, Hannah's drawing is of the mother and baby. The silhouettes lovingly embracing in a spotlight of illumination. This brightness fades into orange, red and then black. The darkness surrounding the warm glow of motherhood is a representation of the ever-present threat. There are also faintly drawn concealed black roots in the image. The roots have the potential to bore into her happiness, but as Hannah exclaimed, 'only if you let them'. The black roots are drawn in pencil and subsequently painted over which could be said to mark a real intent.

The women's images contained unique iconography, and yet interestingly, there were similar messages revealed within their lived experiences. The representations of the light and the dark pervade most of the images. The swirls and movement add energy to the visual depictions, which sometimes portrayed challenging emotional scenarios. It is also important to mention that the study focused on a non-clinical sample, who did not identify as having postnatal mental health difficulties. The next section discusses the themes further and incorporates the mothers' narratives.

Theme 1: The 'Mammy Worry'

All the co-researchers felt what could be described as the 'mammy worry'. In this context, 'mammy worry' is fed by existential concerns and questions. A new mother is thrown into new experiences and senses not only her shifting horizons and possibilities but also that of her child. Concern for her baby's future lies at the core of her experiences; she envisions her baby as a little part of herself wandering the world, naively exploring and experiencing everything with a sense of openness and vulnerability, always trusting. Such innocence has its perils and can give rise to existential fears. On another existential level, mothers can feel alone in bearing responsibility for another life—hence, the 'mammy worry'.

The images all revealed a sense of what it was like for each of the mothers to reflect on their experience of motherhood. The mothers confronted their existence through their babies. The darkness of fear, angst and death became more prominent once their babies arrived. For example, Maggie recounted a distressing and challenging time as a new mother:

> I remember when he was born, and they suspected septicaemia. I remember thinking that I can either go one way or another and I can either be calm about this… or else I can just be hysterical. I cried once in intensive care, but then after that, I just really calmed down. (Maggie)

When faced with her precious baby's mortality, Maggie reasons with her contrasting experience and pivots between 'being calm' and being 'hysterical'. Remarkably, despite the angst, the intensity of her 'mammy worry' put things into perspective, as Maggie admits: 'that kind of anxiety and stuff is still there, whereas other things I just don't care about too much'.

Sarah had a similar experience on becoming a mother and recalled her sorrow at being unable to connect with her daughter on a physical level:

> That was really frightening because I couldn't hold her or take her. So, I spent the whole time sitting over the incubator, crying. I said to myself… it's my fault. (Sarah)

Her formidable and 'frightening' worry instilled a sense of deep fear, which underpinned the unmentionable for Sarah, the possibility that 'she (could) die on me'. Sarah's narrative is imbued with responsibility and possibility. Unfortunately, at that moment loss seems as though it was the only possibility. By the same token, Danielle, Grace, Rebecca and Maggie also imagined worst-case scenarios, as illustrated by the following excerpts:

> It's something that surfaces at times. It's like going into this bottomless pit of darkness, and my mind starts to spiral, and I start thinking about the worst-case scenario. This is what's going to happen. He's going to die. (Danielle)

> I felt that it was going to affect my baby or that she was not going to be able to walk properly (brief pause)... In your mind, you just create such pictures, which are really bad pictures of what could happen. (Grace)

> I'd be fearful that if someone was smoking and they walked past us; that they would infect her. Also, when we were in the car... I would think that cars were going to hit us. (Rebecca)

> It's those senses of anxiety. I think I might be one of those catastrophic thinkers. I jump to the very end. I really have to pull back. But it's all associated with the protection I suppose. (Maggie)

The mother's emotions are ensnared by their future projections, which describe the indescribable; expressions such as 'bottomless pit of darkness', 'spiralling' and 'catastrophic' highlight the uncertainty of their experience concerning their babies. It is evident that the mothers often jump ahead and imagine the worst for their babies, with statements such as 'he's going to die', '(it's) going to hit us' materialising in their narratives. Conversely, Grace upholds that a mother imagines the worst, by creating 'bad pictures', and places the worry firmly within her control.

Irrespective of the influences for these underlying fears, they often inspire watchful behaviours on the mothers' part. For example, Rebecca explains that it is 'this constant worry that something might happen, or you wake up in the middle of the night, and you think, is she breathing?'. Daisy similarly also recalled being vigilant, staying up to watch her son sleep.

> And when he's sleeping, I'm watching him...hands up, I have to admit it. I think I've gone a bit crazy watching him sleeping. (Daisy)

As highlighted from their narratives, the mothers recognised their baby's extreme vulnerabilities. Their fear often centred on something negative happening to their babies and in a bid to protect, some mothers felt the need to stay close to their babies. This ultimately cost them some of their freedom, but this was a choice they made actively.

Theme 2: The Existential Shift of Emotions

The mothers' accounts of their emotional tone and energy were varied and were represented by a spectrum of feeling. Often, they described emotions as unexpected, intense and overwhelming. These emotions were not necessarily specific to people or events and could be situational or non-situational, so could appear to be random, unexplainable and surprising. All the co-researchers noted the intensity and flux of emotions. Moods as described in narrative interviews and as represented in visual images could not be described in simple terms; instead, moods were most often mixed, containing a spectrum of mood and emotions including positive and negative affects.

The moods of motherhood are described as intention-less, being much more diffuse than specific emotions tied to experience. They are also always in flux, moving and shifting, with some mothers talking about their intensity. For example, Danielle eloquently describes the light and dark parts of her image in terms of her experience.

> So, this is me with my baby (pointing to drawing of mother and baby). I suppose it kind of represents the two sides or the different sides that I've been experiencing. The different feelings that I've been going through and the different emotions. A lot of positive represented with the brighter colours and some things don't have any meaning particularly, it's just colours and images I suppose. And as you can tell, this is the negative…the darkest part of what I've been experiencing. (points to the image of the naked figure, in the prone position, crying a river of blood)

Danielle recognises 'the two sides' of her emotional experience, the positive and negative. The darkest part of her experience is vividly depicted as a naked, bald women crying a river of blood. This figure represents her emotional and physical struggle with breastfeeding. The brighter parts are represented with colour, and an image of the mother and babe. Danielle further reflects on the textures she used in the pictures as representing the complexity of motherhood and mood: 'just different textures. Maybe again, representing the complexity of those things and moods that are different'.

Similarly, Rebecca's picture also contains juxtaposing light and dark symbolism. Her image depicts the 'vortex of emotion', with bright dots representing happy moments among the darkness. While Rebecca clarifies the images and the symbols within her image, she states that:

> It's brighter here, and then I did the heart to represent the love. I wrote a massive surge of emotions, so love, fear, anxiety and these are like tears, like a tap that I just couldn't turn off. Actually, a bit emotional now even thinking about it. The worry, you never stop worrying.

The visuals of her emotions being like a running tap that cannot be 'turn(ed) off', inference an energy and uncertainty left free to flow. Her feelings can overwhelm her, but perhaps, on the other hand, the 'running tap' allows her to experience her felt-sense emotions, despite her never-ending worry.

When opening up about her picture, Daisy explains that Winnie the Pooh is not coloured in his traditional yellow and blue outfit and discusses her experience of having a baby as follows;

> [The picture] represents the joy of having a baby. But then I was going to do a lot of different colours just representing the moods that go with it. And to be fair, some of them would be fairly black and then lots of blues and yellows. But now, Winnie might not even be yellow. He could be more lavender-ish and greens and probably darker. Not to say I'm depressed, but it's not as easy as people make out.

Like Rebecca, Daisy acknowledges that motherhood is not easy and challenges the normative depiction of motherhood with her vision of Winnie. Her image and interview convey a sense of something uncannily familiar yet different.

Additionally, it was evident that the women often recognised that their feelings were heightened. Maggie, for example, talked about how her moods are exaggerated, commenting:

> I was kind of thinking my moods …are just more intensified than they normally are. You know… It's like I'm fine, but sometimes I can be a little bit emotionally unsettled, like my mood, it changes.

Maggie relays the sense that these moods assail her unexpectedly. In a similar vein, Rebecca comments that: 'it's very much that things were at the depths of despair, and then things were just great'. The women muse over their fluctuating states of *Being*. There is a real sense of unstable energy and a movement of moods from one extreme to the other. This inner flux also finds a physical embodiment. Daisy, for example, describes her moods as 'sizzling in her brain… Because I can feel my head is fried, honestly'. When asked what that was like, Daisy explains: 'Oh, it's hot. It's physically hot' Danielle relays something similar, saying that:

> It's a massive upheaval in your whole body and your whole self. A lot of emotions, feeling lost one second and the next feeling nothing.

Danielle here shares an embodied experience of mood that demands the attention of her 'whole self' and her 'whole body' and yet even when faced with this formidable energy, she can still feel 'nothing'.

Discussion of the Two Themes

It is evident from the mothers' images and narratives that their worry and fear come from a place of love and care. The tensions which are experienced are balanced by the 'brighter' moments, that assuages their reminders of existence and finitude. In summary, the 'mammy worry' broadly encompasses the mothers' feelings of fear and worry but is fastened to the experience of finitude. Within the co-researchers' narratives, it is often linked to existence itself and the fear of adverse events happening to their most precious babes. All the worries wrapped up in an interconnected bundle of love for their baby. Whereas, the 'existential shift of emotion' represented a more diffuse feeling, a hue of feeling, representing the spectrum of emotions, but did not necessarily have a specific source. It was often expressed as swirls of movement in the images, conveying the overall impression of reaching out and moving towards what they value. Interestingly both angst and mood, from an existential point of view manifest as movement, and if one tunes into the movement and feelings, it can be used as a ladder for greater understanding of self, others and the world.

From the existential perspective, the findings from the study highlight a spectrum of emotions and support the assumption that living and *Being* in the world means welcoming all experiences as well as recognising the transience of feelings. If a mother's mood—or indeed, her mental health—is placed in a category or on a continuum, then that person is imagined as '*Being in*' one place. Nevertheless, the existential self is always in a state of becoming. Consider a mother's emotional self instead as akin to the topographical shape of a Mobius strip, with light and dark as shades of well-being always related, never fixed and ever unfolding. When one is open to the unfolding experiences of *Being*, a change in position or outlook can arise through a process of wondering and reflection. This receptiveness can tilt the edges of our understanding of the mobius-self and illuminate that which was in darkness.

The Mobius strips as seen in Fig. 14.2 are reflective of the current research's findings and are here formed as interlocking hearts, to recognise that the mothers' emotional wavering arises from a place of love and care. It is, moreover, a single band with an interlinking heart reflecting the truth that although a mother's emotions are always in flux, even the dark side of experience has a brighter counterpart around every twist and turn.

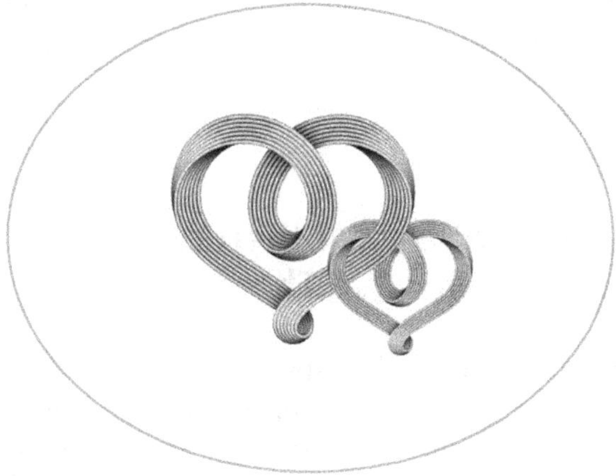

Fig. 14.2 Mobius Hearts of Motherhood (Gaffney 2020)

The findings of this study raise vital questions regarding how we conceptualise and frame first-time mothers' emotional experiences. The findings, while on a sample of women who do not identify as having any diagnosable postnatal mental health difficulties, contribute knowledge to the gap in the literature on mental health and/or well-being in motherhood. It highlights the normative difficulties, which encompass the spectrum of experiences, which were often represented as the bright and dark experiences of *Being* a new mother. The findings also contribute new knowledge and highlight the need for a reflective pause regarding the mothers' well-being, as mothers who are diagnosed with perinatal mental health difficulties are not always given a chance to reflect on their emotional experiences, nor are such answers or reflections counted in formal diagnosis.

Many of the co-researchers seem to have benefited from the opportunity to explore their thoughts and feelings as part of the image creation and interview process, with Sarah mentioning that 'she really enjoyed the experience'. Danielle and Grace both stated they liked creating the image even though it was difficult to know where to begin. Grace remarked that it was nice to have the time to herself to complete the image. The mothers profited from having time to reflect, as well as being offered a specific theme to consider. This aspect is considered in the next section, as the findings also support a practical engagement with mothers from a therapeutic perspective. At this point, it is worth noting that the methodology described has the potential for application to parenthood experiences from different vantage points and could be extended upon with further research.

Practical Application: Motherhood and Existential Creative Therapy

Existential psychotherapy and art psychotherapy practices have many similarities. Both practices are interested in the opening up of the client's possibilities. Both Existential Therapy and Art Therapy recognise the uniqueness of each person's experience and the idiographic meaning systems created in a therapy session. Existential Creative Therapy can capture the paradoxes and the tensions of existence on paper and provide an alternative or complementary way to confront the ultimate concerns of human existence: death, freedom, existential isolation and meaninglessness (Yalom 1980). Art offers a unique channel for asking and answering ontological questions and confronting existential challenges. For example, Bruce Moon (2007) devised a version of Existential Art Therapy that invited clients to process their dreams through artmaking. He emphasised the autonomy that artistic processes afford. Moon celebrated the inherent freedom of the art. He concluded that an arts-based approach helps people create meaning from chaos and confusion, perhaps defining the existential drive behind the intrinsic human impulse to make art. Besides, creative methods can enhance and sometimes work around the shortcomings of language by utilising a pictorial language. Confronting one's existence with the use of a pictorial language can enrich research and therapeutic discussions because it is said to be akin to a pre-verbal form of communication (Vasarhelyi 1981, 2002). When explaining the image created, a mother has time to reflect on her experience before verbalising its meaning. Existential-focused enquiry enables the mother to develop her pictorial vocabulary and unique iconography. No external interpretation needs to be superimposed on a person's visual language. Instead, an existential visual enquiry can help tease out understandings and meanings related to the mother's worldview.

The Four Dimensions

A new mother navigating her way through her experience will confront four dimensions of existence: Umwelt, Mitwelt, Eigenwelt, and Uberwelt (Binswanger 1946, 1963; van Deurzen 1988). (This has been discussed in detail in Chapters 2 and 15). In the next section, the four dimensions form a framework of understanding when utilising creativity in existential practice.

An Existential Opening for Creative Practice

Creating an image can be a daunting experience that requires a willingness to reflect deeply on oneself and can ultimately reveal questions about one's existence. The process of drawing can mirror the new lives of mother and child insofar as- all involve creation. Tillich (1952) discussed the tension and the uncomfortable in the creative process, which he compared to the need for self-understanding and the desire to apprehend one's relationship with the external world. Merleau-Ponty (1964) also viewed art in this way and argued that art was an inter-subjective engagement with the world. Thus, artmaking is both an inter-subjective and an intra-subjective activity.

The main themes discussed by the mothers intimated a confrontation with existence. Ontological questions such as: Who am I as a mother? and Who am I as a member of a family? were realised. Existential shifts in one's experience can fuel the 'mammy worry' and inspire fears about managing motherhood. To begin revealing these moods and emotions, themes can be provided for exploration. These themes can be utilised in individual or group sessions. These themes are derived directly from my research study, my training in Art Therapy (Vasarhelyi Method) and my professional practice (Table 14.1).

In keeping with phenomenological existential practice, Existential Creative Therapy requires therapists to be aware of themselves when working with the mother (client) and her image. The process requires *Attention*, awareness of *Epoché* and *Verification.* The creation of the image necessitates the client—in this case, the mother—to take some time to create what she would like to share in the session. The following steps can be followed.

1. **Start of the Session**: Once the session has begun and rapport with the mother is established, the therapist should allow the mother time to complete the image and should sit outside the room for an agreed time frame (20–30 minutes) while the image is completed (Vasarhelyi 1981, 2002). The underlying idea is that the mother should have the time and space required without being conscious or aware of the therapist.

Table 14.1 Existential art themes

General Themes	Questions	Themes (derived from the research study)
Self	Create an image of yourself, while reflecting on how you see yourself?	Who am I?
Family	Create an image of your family, while reflecting on how you see them?	Becoming a family
Important experiences	Create an image of your experience of motherhood? It can be an experience that is on your mind that you would like to share?	The unexpected and surprises of motherhood
Worry	Create an image of an area/areas in your life that create tensions or worries for you?	The 'mammy worry'
Phenomenon of feeling	Create an image of how you feel. And while you are creating the image, think about your mood and emotions?	Emotional tensions/experiences
Coping skills	How do you manage *Being* a mother? Create an image of your coping strategies?	Managing motherhood

2. **The Therapist Returns**: When the therapist re-enters the room, she/he will see the image for the first time; this reaction will create an original response. The phenomenological practice of *Attention* is employed as an essential starting point in all therapeutic engagement. Once the therapist sees the image, it is natural that one's attention is drawn to the familiar. This is what can be called an original response; however, the therapist should attend and observe and thus, *Epoché* is essential. *Epoché* the suspension of judgement and the bracketing of assumptions.
3. **Gaining Description**: The mother should be invited to tell the therapist about the image in as much detail as possible. Again, the practice of *Epoché* is valuable as the therapist should listen to what the image means to the mother.

4. **The Clarification and Verification Process**: The *verification* process contains a hermeneutic function, which is to understand the mother's meaning within the image. This process can include *clarification* and *verification* of one's understanding of the meaning within the image in keeping with what is called *horizontalization*: the placing of what is becoming known, against a horizon, thus, in this instance contextualising the mothers' worldview.
5. **Clarifying Questions**: One's *attention* and further requests for description are essential as an engagement with the philosophical and the creative. *Clarifying* questions can be asked, and meanings discussed to help tie together the various aspects (van Deurzen & Adams 2011: 43). The four worlds can provide an existential framework for greater depth of understanding. This aspect is outlined briefly in the next section.

The following descriptive table was formulated initially for dream analysis (ibid.: 98–99), with additional questions added regarding emotion and creativity. It can be used within the session, or similarly, it can be applied after the session to tease out meaning. It is not a chronological list of questions; instead, it provides an existential framework for reviewing images systematically and was utilised in the previously outlined research study as an aid for analysis and understanding. As a result, aspects of the table can be used at the therapist's discretion (Table 14.2).

Expected Outcomes

There is no set outcome of the exploration, but it can be hoped that the mother will feel safe and secure to explore the tensions within her experiences and understand her mode of *Being-in-the-World* as a mother. Moreover, by providing the time and engaging in existential enquiries, the possible paradoxes and dilemmas will come to the fore. The mother's strengths and weaknesses may be revealed along with existential meanings that inspire a deeper level of reflection. The concepts of understanding and un-concealment are linked to the process of Existential Creative Therapy. I believe that this individual progression involves

Table 14.2 The four dimensions: A creative investigative tool

World	Analysis of drawing
Physical Umwelt	1. What is represented in the image? (natural or human-made objects?)
	2. Describe the objects, the animals, the creatures in the image?
	3. Are the images or symbols known or unknown to the creator?
	4. Are there sensations/embodied experiences in the image?
	5. Is the physical world safe for the mother and child?
	6. Is there interaction with the bodies of others?
	7. What are the risks, the threats to physical existence for the mother and child? How are they encountered?
Social Mitwelt	1. Is the mother/figure(s) alone, or connected?
	2. How many others are there? Are they close, familiar, or distant?
	3. Are they friendly or threatening, helpful or dangerous?
	4. What are the social roles the mother has in the image?
	5. Is she active, passive, proactive or helpless in relation to others?
	6. Is there co-operation and a sense of community present, or is there a sense of hostility and or threat?
	7. Is there love, or an aspiration to love?
	8. What is the threat and promise of others? How does the mother encounter this?
Personal Eigenwelt	1. What is the personal world saying in the drawing to the mother?
	2. Does she have a clear sense of identity and recognition of this identity? i.e. is she prominent or absent?
	3. Does the mother know what she wants?
	4. What character traits are sketched out-through the actions of the image: e.g. courage or cowardice, intelligence or stupidity, self-reliance or need of others?
	5. Is the person in the image kind, harsh, understanding, intolerant, supportive or challenging to herself?
	6. What are her intentions, desires and objectives? Is she aware of these?

(continued)

Table 14.2 (continued)

World	Analysis of drawing
Spiritual Uberwelt	1. What sort of world does the mother believe she lives in?
	2. How is the mother situated in this visual world? i.e. What is her worldview?
	3. What is it that makes the image meaningful?
	4. Are her wishes and desires evident or expressed?
	5. What are the values, assumptions, beliefs and principles conveyed?
	6. Are her morals or ethics prominent?
	7. What is it for the mother that really matters at the end of the day, and what stands in the way of achieving this?
	8. What is the implied purpose in the image?
Emotions	1. What was your mood like when... happened?
	2. How did you experience this? What was that like for you?
	3. What emotions came up for you when you reflected on...?
Themes	1. What themes or patterns does the mother notice or recognise?
	2. How do these themes reflect her life in the here and now?
	3. What aspects are prominent for her in the image (what did it reveal to her)?
Creative Practice	1. What was the experience of creating the image like? 2. Discuss the mother's choice of colour and medium.

a process of unfolding and becoming, which is likened to Heraclitus' (c. 540–480–BC) flowing river, never static and always becoming. In this view, embracing rather than resisting change as a mother; will generate fresh inspiration (Howard 2000).

Conclusion

Becoming a mother entails a shift in experience and emotion, wherein a new mother is faced frankly with her own and her baby's existence. Motherhood involves questions of life and death about herself and her baby that give rise to strong emotions. The research studies findings show that strong fluctuating emotions and heightened fears and anxieties are part of the 'normal' experience of motherhood. Mothers selflessly give to their babies without question and with an immense amount of joy and love. Nevertheless, love often comes with much physical, psychological and emotional pain, as mothers question themselves and their abilities. However, such experiences in motherhood are rarely discussed normatively.

An existential psychology framework and a existential creative framework de-pathologise the moods of motherhood to support a mother's reflection on her own experience. This approach contrasts with the current mainstream applications for motherhood and mood by nurturing matters of meaning, purpose, choice, responsibility and relationships while recognising the paradoxes and tensions of existence without judgement.

References

Binswanger, L. (1946 [1958]). The Existential Analysis School of Thought. In R. May, E Angel, & H. F. Ellenberger (Eds.), *Existence*. New York: Basic Books.

Binswanger, L. (1963). *Being-in-the-World*. Trans. J. Needleman. New York: Basic Books.

Heidegger, M. (1962 [1927]). *Being and Time*. Trans. J. Macquarrie & E. Robinson. New York, NY: Harper & Row.
Howard, A. (2000). *Philosophy for Counselling and Psychotherapy: Pythagoras to Postmodernism*. Basingstoke: Palgrave.
Kierkegaard, S. (2015 [1844]). *The Concept of Anxiety*. Trans. A. Hannay. London: Liverlight.
Merleau-Ponty, M. (1964). *The Primacy of Perception: And Other Essays on Phenomenological Psychology, the Philosophy of Art, History, and Politics*. Evanston, IL: Northwestern University Press.
Moon, B. L. (2007). Dialoguing with Dreams in Existential Art Therapy. *Art Therapy, 24*(3), 128–133. https://doi.org/10.1080/07421656.2007.10129428.
Tillich, P. (2000 [1952]). *The Courage to Be* (2nd ed.). New Haven, CT: Yale University Press.
van Deurzen, E. (1988). *Existential Counselling in Practice*. London: Sage.
van Deurzen, E. (2009). *Everyday Mysteries: A Handbook of Existential Psychotherapy*. London: Routledge.
van Deurzen, E., & Adams, M. (2011). *Skills in Existential Counselling & Psychotherapy* (2nd ed.). London: Sage.
Vasarhelyi, V. (1981). What Happened on Ben Nevis? Psychotherapy with Pictorial Means and the Time Aspect of Pictorial Thinking. *Special Study-Goldsmith's College* (pp 27–45). London: Goldsmiths.
Vasarhelyi, V. (2002). The Cat, the Fish, the Man, and the Bird: Or How to Be a Nothing. Illness Behaviour in Children; The Case Study of a 10-Year-Old Girl. In *Working with Children in Art Therapy*. London: Routledge.
Yalom, I. D. (1980). *Existential Psychotherapy*. New York, NY: Basic Books.

15

Existential Group Work with Mothers

Claire Arnold-Baker and Victoria Garland

Introduction

An inherent part of being human is that we are social beings. Heidegger termed this '*being-with*' (Heidegger 1962), to denote that we are always in relationship with others. It is crucial to note the importance others can have on our experiences, our mental health and our ability to cope with the challenges we must face in life. In fact, evolutionary anthropologists have highlighted that the social aspect of childbirth is what sets us apart from other mammals. The fact that others provide intense emotional and physical support to birthing mothers is an aspect that makes us human (Rosenberg 2012). However, this support is not just needed during the time of childbirth but extends out into the first year of the baby's life. Stern recognised the importance of the support new mothers needed and included a supporting-matrix theme to his concept of the motherhood

C. Arnold-Baker · V. Garland (✉)
The New School of Psychotherapy and Counselling, London, UK

C. Arnold-Baker
e-mail: claire@nspc.org.uk

C. Arnold-Baker (ed.), *The Existential Crisis of Motherhood*,
https://doi.org/10.1007/978-3-030-56499-5_15

constellation. He understood the 'mother's need to create, permit, accept, and regulate a protecting, benign support network' (Stern 1995: 177), one which the mother could create herself but also one that was created for the mother by those who cared for her. Stern felt that this support network was essential for the mother if she was able to keep her baby alive and protect its psychic development. He saw two functions of the support-matrix. The first was to protect the mother physically and attend to her needs, certainly in the early stages of motherhood. The second function of the matrix was to provide the mother with psychological and educational support. However, sadly this level of support is not universally available to Western women and certainly not formally structured in ways that would be found in other cultures where women are given support whilst they adjust to their new role and experience (Kruckman 1992).

Maternal Support

Research into maternal support has found that those mothers who had good support networks generally coped better than those without. Price noted that those 'women who survive the traumas of disillusionment with the social experience of mothering best are those who have close, non-critical relationships with other women' (Price 1988: 22). Collins et al. (1993) found that mothers who had good social support during the birth experienced a better progress through labour. They concluded that social support may reduce the extent to which situations are seen as stressful. Goldstein et al. (1996) found that those mothers who had a larger support network were more sensitive in their interactions with their baby. Further research conducted by Cronin (2003) demonstrated the importance of the maternal mother in helping first-time mothers adapt to their new roles and responsibilities. Social support therefore seems critical to the mother's ability to cope.

Social support also gives the mother an opportunity to gather information (Stern 1995; Stadlen 2005; Arnold-Baker 2015). Stadlen noted that cooperative links with other mothers were vital and tended to focus on immediate practical questions concerning the care of the baby. But the importance of adult company should not be discounted, as Arnold-Baker (2015) found, adult company and conversation gave mothers a sense of normality and a link back to the adult world that they were familiar with. Informational support and appraisal has also been found to positively influence the confidence of first-time mothers in their infant care practices (Warren 2005).

Price documents how often depression is missed by health visitors and GPs because it creeps up on a mother. She also highlights anxiety as another form of distress that is often missed. New mothers often feel overwhelming anxiety which 'reflects a complex mixture of a heightened awareness of the real dangers of the external world, which suddenly seem to be all around, and also of the dangers internally' (Price 1988: 138–139). For Price then motherhood, particularly in the first year, leaves a woman '… psychologically vulnerable. Her physical resources are continuously drained with little time for respite and her psychological boundaries are breeched in a way that makes her vulnerable to any hint of criticism' (ibid.: 141). Price believes that women most able to cope psychologically to motherhood are those who are realistic about the expectations of being a mother and honest about their experience and who are supported by like-minded women.

Finding like-minded women is crucial if mothers are to be able to talk openly and honestly about their experiences. Mothers who were able to participate in an open exchange with others who were in the same position as themselves were also able to provide mutual support (Arnold-Baker 2015). The mothers in Arnold-Baker's study, who were successful professionals prior to becoming mothers, were able to be open about their experiences with each other and not as Maushart (1999) suggested, hiding behind the 'mask of silence'. This suggested that when mothers feel able to trust other mothers they can be open about their 'bad' days and of 'not knowing'. When mothers do not feel supported or unable to find like-minded mothers, then it seems they resort to 'the mask of motherhood' and keep their true experiences of motherhood to themselves. Most of the mothers in Arnold-Baker's research belonged to support groups such as the NCT (National Childbirth Trust). Being part of a group which met regularly before the baby was born did seem to be helpful for the mothers in developing good and trusting relationships with the other mothers in their group, and this enabled them to share some of what they were experiencing with each other. One of the mothers interviewed described how this had made a big difference to her and that she would have found meeting and bonding with mothers after the birth more difficult. Interestingly, another participant in this research mentioned how she wasn't able to bond with one of the mothers in her NCT group who seemed to have a 'perfect' baby. She felt that this mother, who had the 'easy' baby, was not going through the same experiences and difficulties that she and the other members of the group were going through, and this created a distance between them. This highlights that not all groups are necessarily supportive, and women tend to search for other women who have shared similar experiences to themselves. NCT groups, for example, despite being open to all often attracts mothers who are, predominately white, heteronormative and middle-class, and therefore, these groups might not appeal to all women. Therefore, it is important to create support groups where women feel accepted and supported and where a range of maternal experiences are acknowledged and valued.

Re-Setting and Support

The mothers in Arnold-Baker's research described how meeting regularly with other mothers 're-set' or distracted them, so that any difficulty they were facing at that moment appeared less and it gave them the strength to carry on despite these difficulties. Although not all mothers experience depression, most will find being a new mother hard. As Beth described, there were times when she 'wanted to hide under the duvet' (Arnold-Baker 2015: 111). This notion of re-setting described how the mothers were able to put their difficulties behind them and it felt like they were starting again, with renewed strength. This finding demonstrated how by sharing their experiences the mothers were able to normalise them and get a sense of perspective on their situation. But they also needed, as Price found 'a sense of being heard and understood, to validate our own experience' (Price 1988: 142). Connecting with other mothers also meant that they felt less isolated as they knew there was a point in the week when they could meet up with their group and share what had been going on for them. Other research, (Goldstein et al. 1996; Collins et al. 1993) found that social support, if it was found to be satisfactory by the mother, did reduce the extent to which circumstances were viewed as stressful. Goldstein et al. found that mothers with large social networks had more opportunity to have their needs met and were therefore more able to meet the needs of their babies.

The process of re-setting involved several aspects. The first was that the participants were able to 'hold' their difficult feelings and experiences because they knew there was a time and place for them to talk through those feelings. It allowed them to keep going even in the darkest of times because there was an anchor point ahead. The second aspect involved talking about, sharing and listening to other mothers' experiences. This helped the mothers to normalise their experience but also to see that others were also struggling, sometimes in different ways. This enabled the mothers to begin to see there was no one way to be a mother and that each mother needed to find their own way with their baby. They described how meeting up also offered a distraction, so that their attention was taken away from the minutiae of looking after their babies and they became less absorbed in the world of their babies. This all helped the mothers to put their own experiences and difficulties into perspective. Having gained this new perspective, they were able to put these feelings and experiences in the past and to move forward. The mothers were able to start again from that point, anew; the difficulties they had been experiencing now seemed less overpowering and overwhelming. Through this process, they had gained some strength and felt they were more able to continue and cope with the demands of motherhood.

Existential Group Work

The evidence from previous research on the importance of support for mothers is overwhelming and yet mothers are often unable to access the type of support that they need. Whilst some mothers will reach out for individual support provided by a therapist or a health professional, this can also seem a daunting prospect for many. The need for postnatal support groups seems imperative. As the chapters in this book have shown, a group based on existential principles will enable mothers to engage with the momentaneous changes that have occurred since their babies were born.

Existential groups create a safe space for each member to have the time and the freedom to talk through their difficulties, to hear about the struggles of others, to become aware of how they respond to others in the group and to experiment with new ways of being. The group enables the participants to enter into real relationships with each other and the group is facilitated in such a way that it is fair and respectful but also that the facilitator is genuine in their interactions (Tantam and van Deurzen 2019).

The normal parameters of groups, such as time and space, are important. The facilitator needs to ensure that the sessions start and end on time but also take into account how time is taken up in the group. The facilitator will note how the time is divided between the group members or how much time is spent on individual issues compared to issues of the group itself. Taking account of these issues of time ensures that each member feels safe and that they can take up group time when they need to.

It is also important to create the group space so that it is one that feels safe and that members want to be a part of and contribute to. The facilitator holds an important role here in modelling respectful listening to each other. Group members will learn more about themselves if they are able to be self-reflective and gain supportive feedback from their peers. Facilitators will discuss with group members how they can keep themselves safe in the group and consider the impact of their disclosures for themselves and for others.

Group facilitators will also need to be mindful of the new mothers' needs. Most likely mothers will attend the group carrying their babies, and mothers may need to feed them or soothe them when they are crying. These are issues to consider as well as the potential impact they may have on the other members of the group. In addition, new mothers may not be able to give the group their full commitment depending on the needs of their babies.

The framework for the perinatal support group has an existential focus which has been developed out of our research and work with mothers. The chapters of this book have shown the many existential issues that new mothers face after the birth of their babies. Enabling women to reflect on these issues has been found to be helpful for processing and making sense of their motherhood experiences. By highlighting the universal aspects of our existence that are present in motherhood helps to normalise the mothers' experiences and offers a non-pathological way of understanding the tremendous changes that have occurred.

A defining feature of an existential approach to therapy is the holistic view it takes of the individual. It stresses the importance of each individual's personal context. We cannot escape the fact that we are situational, and that we live in a world which has certain constraints and limitations. Nor can we assume that every person will react and respond in the same ways to the circumstances that they find themselves in. However, through using the four dimensions of existence as a framework and guide, mothers can reflect on the ways in which they interact with the world and others and with themselves and how this might have changed after childbirth.

Four Dimensions of Existence—Umwelt, Mitwelt, Eigenwelt and Überwelt

The four dimensions of existence developed out of Heidegger's (1962) concept of Being-in-the-world, and his view that we are not isolated subjects but exist as *being-with*. May (1983) clarified Binswanger's (1963) initial world views to describe the four basic dimensions of human existence.

The *Umwelt* therefore represents the world that we are thrown into. *Thrownness* is Heidegger's concept to describe the way in which we belong to a world that existed before our birth and over which we have no control. This world includes our relationship to our physical environment; it is also the world of our biological drives, impulses, senses and our awareness of our body and our bodily needs. The *Umwelt* would also encompass our physical sense of space, the space we take up but also the space around us.

The *Mitwelt*, however, represents the social dimension of existence. This aspect highlights our rational nature with others, both friends and family but also other people that we meet and interact with in our lives. This dimension also includes the other ways in which we relate socially, such as to our culture, our society and to our language.

The *Eigenwelt* concerns the world of the self or the personal dimension. This dimension is about our relationship with our sense of self and our relationships with intimate others. It also includes our feelings, thoughts and character traits. The *Eigenwelt* is where human beings create a sense of who they are.

A fourth dimension of existence, the *Überwelt*, was added by van Deurzen (2010) and represents the spiritual dimension. This dimension represents the world of our values and beliefs, our ideal world. It is the dimension in which we create meaning and find purpose and make sense of our lives.

Each dimension contains its own paradoxes and challenges, which highlight different aspects and existential issues. Our research has shown that motherhood is complex and comprised of multi-layered experiences which are intertwined and interrelated across the four dimensions of existence. Further, the transition to motherhood is an existential crisis which reveals a transformative journey that begins when a woman leaves the familiar world she knew before and finds herself in the unknown world of motherhood.

Existential Framework for Perinatal Support Groups

The existential framework that is suggested in this chapter will guide mothers through each dimension, providing a space for them to reflect on the challenges and paradoxes that they have faced during their transition to motherhood and to see the uniqueness and the commonality of their experiences. This framework allows for diverse motherhood experiences as each mother can reflect on her own journey, context and experience within the four dimensions.

Furthermore, addressing the transition to motherhood as an existential crisis instead of a pathological one encourages women to view motherhood as a life event that mobilises self-reflection through existential questioning.

Framework for a 14-Week Group

This short-term structured group was designed to allow mothers to have an opportunity to explore the immense changes that occur during their transition to motherhood. The four dimensions of existence provide an existential theoretical frame to guide mothers during their explorations. Through understanding their transition in existential terms, mothers will be given the opportunity to gain a better self-awareness and through self-growth find a more mindful and authentic way of living.

Proposed structure for a 14-week perinatal support group:

Week 1 Introductions, expectations and setting ground rules
Weeks 2–4 Exploration of the physical dimension
Weeks 5–7 Examining relationships within the social dimension
Weeks 8–10 Focussing on the personal dimension
Weeks 11–13 Finding meaning within the spiritual dimension
Week 14 Conclusion and feedback.

To enable each mother to have enough space and time to reflect and talk about their experiences, a two-hour weekly format is suggested for between 6 and 8 mothers. Table 15.1 summarises the areas that facilitators can explore with mothers to ensure that they are able to reflect on all aspects of their motherhood journey.

Table 15.1 Areas of existential exploration for existential groups with mothers

Dimension	Areas of existential exploration
Physical	Embodied nature of motherhood—pregnancy, birth and breastfeeding Sexuality and the sexual body Life and death Time Lack of sleep and exhaustion
Social	Renegotiating relationship with their partner Reflection and revisiting relationship with their own mother Loss of old connections Gaining new friendships Judgements of others: 'good mother'
Personal	Changes to the mother's sense of self Feelings of responsibility Personal choices and choices for the baby Emotional response: anxiety, guilt, intense love, frustration
Spiritual	Re-evaluation and reorganisation of values New meanings emerge Purpose in life changes Spiritual connection of the mother–child relationship Spiritual growth of the mother

Introduction Session

The initial session allows mothers to introduce themselves and for the facilitator to introduce the theoretical framework. The facilitator needs to use accessible words and phrases when explaining what the physical, social, personal and spiritual dimensions represent. The setting of ground rules and expectations are also equally important as well as creating a safe, collaborative space for mothers.

The Exploration of Physical Dimension

By placing a focus on the embodied nature of motherhood, women can reflect on how their bodies have changed during pregnancy, labour or after the birth. Often mothers feel there is no place for them to talk about these experiences however, in a group they can find a space to reflect on their often traumatic experiences of labour, to process those experiences, to be heard and to feel that they matter too.

Motherhood also confronts women with the possibilities and limitations of their embodiment. Mothers describe a high level of anxiety when faced with the fragility of their children and mothers can be guided to reflect on the unpredictability of life and death and what that means for them and the way they think about their lives.

Physical exhaustion is also a major issue that mothers face, both from a lack of sleep but also a psychological exhaustion from the all-encompassing nature of motherhood. Mothers' experience of time and the structure of their day change too, leading them to feel out of control when they feel they need to be organised. The ever-present sense of responsibility which keeps the mothers focussed on their babies at every moment also creates a tiredness, as mothers are always on alert. This level of tiredness, both physical and psychological, comes as a shocking surprise to most mothers.

Mothers may also talk about how they feel about their bodies. Some mothers may describe how proud they are of what they have achieved, others may feel let down by their bodies if they had a difficult labour or were unable to breastfeed. Some mothers may feel lucky to 'get back' to their previous shape, whereas often women feel unhappy about their bodies and not in control of how they have changed. Facilitators can help mothers reflect on how their female bodies become a kind of 'currency' that is used for acceptance and integration 'back' into society in the postnatal period. Or how they express or feel about their sexuality and gender postnatally.

The Exploration of Social Dimension

In giving birth to a child, a mother gives birth to new relationships, to her baby but also to her partner. Parents go from being a couple to a family, and however close and tender their relationships were before having children, mothers are often surprised to feel more separate following the birth of their child. Often it takes time for them to reconnect with their partner. Parents are often unprepared for this change from coupledom to family life and how they will need to assimilate each other's views and family backgrounds to be able to create their own way of being a family.

Mothers may also be drawn to revisiting their relationships with their own mothers. Sometimes a new understanding is found, or mothers choose to emulate or distance themselves from the mothering they received as a child.

Women often describe the loss of old connections but also how they have gained new friendships. Their social lives are less flexible now and they become less available to their previous friendships. However, mothers are also gaining new connections with other mothers with whom they can share their experiences, feel understood, comforted, reassured and affirmed in their unfamiliar roles as mothers.

Facilitators can enable mothers to become aware that they are making different choices and prioritising different aspects of their social world. Finding like-minded mothers can help mothers feel less isolated, less anxious and more reassured in making choices and taking on their responsibilities. However, this is by no means without its challenges as mothers describe how they also compare themselves to other mothers.

Mothers share a strong awareness of feeling judged by others, both for their own and their child's actions, as they try to conform to societal norms and expectations. Often discussions about feeding raise these feelings and mothers often express feeling like a 'Bad mother' if they did not breastfeed their babies.

Facilitators could encourage mothers to reflect on how socially constructed concepts of 'Good' or 'Bad' mother have moulded their own evaluation of their mothering abilities. Therefore, it is important for mothers to share their experiences and gain self-confidence and acceptance of being 'Good enough' mothers.

The Exploration of Personal Dimension

It can be argued that giving birth to a child automatically assigns an identity as mother, but choosing motherhood informs, shapes and develops that identity. A mother's identity is created therefore through her relationship with herself, her experiences and her relationships with others. Some women describe experiencing a loss of a sense of self, whilst others describe changes in the way they see themselves.

Facilitators can help new mothers see that the changes their experience in their sense of themselves are not a loss of identity as such, but a transformation due to the enormous changes that are occurring in their lives. Our sense of who we are comes out of our embodied interactions in the world, but it takes time for mothers to assimilate those changes into a sense of identity.

As a consequence of taking responsibility for their children's well-being, women often describe feelings of high anxiety of wrongdoing, inadequacy and guilt. They describe how caring for their infant involves moral ambiguity over how to best understand and fulfil their babies' needs. However, over time mothers find their own unique mothering style, learning how to respond to their child's needs whilst balancing them with their own needs.

Identity is not a static or solid entity but a process that evolves and transforms with our life experiences and the choices we make. Mothers who return to work need to be able to balance their identity as a mother with the other identities they hold in society, particularly as mothers are confronted with societal discourses which define women as either working mothers or traditional mothers. This in turn demonstrates how our social norms are gendered, that to be a parent and a professional is different for a man and a woman and this creates a challenge for women who face navigating both situations.

Facilitators could help mothers see the unique paradox of their existence of being intensely bound to another, and at the same time being free and separate. They can enable women to gain an understanding of themselves as mothers in their unique situation, not defined by social tropes, and to find their own way of being-in-the-world as mothers.

Reflecting on the Spiritual Dimension

During the exploration of experiences in the spiritual dimension, most mothers express feeling surprised at being overwhelmed by the intensity of their emotional responses to their child. They describe their mother–child relationship as 'unlike any other', a feeling of unconditional love beyond words and impossible to understand unless you have experienced it yourself. Mothers often describe intense feelings of intimacy, a newfound sense of connectedness, interdependence and general relatedness. An example of relational spirituality was demonstrated by one mother who described how the love she had for her child had become an 'awakening' of 'life energy'. Although these intense feelings of love are not felt by all mothers, and certainly not straight away and this can also cause mothers to question themselves if they don't experience the 'rush of love' they had expected to feel.

Furthermore, mothers talk about the re-evaluation and re-organisation of their values and priorities, and how becoming a mother changes their meaning and purpose of life. Mothers find new meaning through their relationships with their children and describe this new meaning as a deep commitment and responsibility for their children's well-being. It could be argued that the spiritual dimension takes the mother–child relationship beyond the relational field and points to a spiritual connection that nurtures not only the growth of the child but also the transformational growth of the mother.

On the spiritual dimension, the facilitator could help new mothers observe how the path mothers take in their journey is paved with 'the unknown' on all four dimensions of existence. Mothers are continually confronted with new situations, new challenges and expectations and are often left feeling unskilled. 'Not knowing', although anxiety provoking, paradoxically allows mothers to be open to their experiences which can lead to new possibilities being available to them.

Concluding Session

The final session invites mothers to reflect on their explorations during the group, to provide feedback and to discuss any questions or worries with the facilitator. This last session is also an opportunity for the mothers to sum up what has been useful and what they will take from the group. Creating a good ending for each of the mothers in the group is also important.

The overall feedback from a number of groups has demonstrated how the exploration of motherhood using the four dimensions of existence as a map can provide facilitators with a comprehensive framework to support mothers in addressing their changes on each dimension. The existential framework allows mothers to explore how the dimensions are interrelated and help them relate those changes to the bigger picture of their new 'Being-in-the-world' as mothers. Enabling mothers to think through the existential issues that come to the fore during motherhood will help them understand themselves and their experience in a deeper way and help them to make more mindful and authentic choices that lead to personal strength and empowerment. Treating motherhood as an existential crisis rather than a pathological one will navigate the focus away from self-criticism and self-blame towards normalising and welcoming their powerful maternal experiences. This places an emphasis on understanding challenges and difficulties rather than seeking to fixing them which has been found to be helpful to mothers seeking to better understand their experiences.

References

Arnold-Baker, C. (2015). How Becoming a Mother Involves a Confrontation with Existence: An Existential-Phenomenological Exploration of the Experience of Early Motherhood. *Degree of Doctor of Counselling Psychology, Middlesex University Repository*.

Binswanger, L. (1963). *Being-in-the-World*. Trans. J. Needleman. New York: Basic Books.

Collins, N. L., Dunkel-Schetter, C., Lobel, M., & Scrimshaw, S. C. M. (1993). Social Support in Pregnancy: Psychosocial Correlates of Birth Outcomes and Postpartum Depression. *Journal of Personality and Social Psychology, 65*(6), 1243–1258.

Cronin, C. (2003). First-time Mothers—Identifying Their Needs, Perceptions and Experiences. *Journal of Clinical Nursing, 12*, 260–267.

Garland, V. (2019). 'Being-in-the-world' as a Mother Hermeneutic-Phenomenological Exploration of Lived Experiences of Eight New Mothers' Transition to Motherhood Within the Theoretical Frame of 'Four Dimensions of Existence.' *Degree of Doctor of Counselling Psychology, Middlesex University Repository.*

Goldstein, L. H., Diener, M. L., & Mangelsdorf, S. C. (1996). Maternal Characteristics and Social Support Across the Transition to Motherhood: Associations with Maternal Behaviour. *Journal of Family Psychology, 10*(1), 60–71.

Heidegger, M. (1962). *Being and Time*. Trans. J. Macquarrie & E. S. Robinson. New York: Harper & Row.

Kruckman, L. D. (1992). Rituals and Support: An Anthropological View of Postpartum Depression. In J. A. Hamilton & P. N. Harberger (Eds.), *Postpartum Psychiatric Illness: A Picture Puzzle*. Philadelphia: University of Pennsylvania.

Maushart, S. (1999). *The Mask of Motherhood*. London: Pandora.

May, R. (1983). *The Discovery of Being*. New York: Norton.

Price, J. (1988). *Motherhood: What It Does to Your Mind*. London: Pandora.

Rosenberg, K. R. (2012). What Makes us Human? Answers from Evolutionary Anthropology. *Evolutionary Anthropology, 21*, 182–194.

Stadlen, N. (2005). *What Mothers Do: Especially When It Looks like Nothing*. London: Piatkus.

Stern, D. (1995). *The Motherhood Constellation: A Unified View of Parent-Infant Psychotherapy*. London: Karnac Books.

Tantam, D., & van Deurzen, E. (2019). Existential Group Therapy: Method and Practice. In E. van Deurzen, et al. (Eds.), *The Wiley World Handbook of Existential Therapy*. Chichester: Wiley.

van Deurzen, E. (2010). *Everyday Mysteries: A handbook of Existential Psychotherapy*. London: Routledge.

Warren, P. L. (2005). First-time Mothers: Social Support and Confidence in Infant Care. *Journal of Advanced Nursing, 50*(5), 479–488.

16

Conclusion: The Courage to Be

Claire Arnold-Baker

A wealth of different motherhood experiences and voices have been brought together in this book; spanning a number of issues that women face as part of their motherhood journey. However, as already stressed at the beginning of the book, this is by no means a definitive list and there are many diverse ways in which women can be mothers. Yet, I would argue that there are core themes that run through these various experiences. Commonalities that all mothers confront regardless of their particular situations. There is the shock or surprise that comes with being a new mum, the sense of the unknown or of not understanding this new experience, and the worry and responsibility that is felt taking care of a vulnerable baby or child. But there are also common existential themes that come to the fore such as choice, responsibility, freedom, mortality, temporality and identity. These are elements that we all face as human beings; however, they come together in such a way during motherhood that it represents an existential crisis for women. These existential aspects

C. Arnold-Baker (✉)
The New School of Psychotherapy and Counselling, London, UK
e-mail: claire@nspc.org.uk

C. Arnold-Baker (ed.), *The Existential Crisis of Motherhood*,
https://doi.org/10.1007/978-3-030-56499-5_16

transcend the uniqueness of each maternal experience as they concern the fundamental conditions of being human.

The chapters in this book have shown how women are confronted by their choices, in a way that throws their whole existence into question. This sense of choice permeates every aspect of motherhood, from choosing to have a baby or not, from accepting being a mother with all that it entails, to the minutiae choices that are part of our everyday existence. These everyday choices that make up our lives are ones we might not even be aware we are making. We make thousands of choices each day, from what to wear or what to eat, to how we respond to others or how we fill our time. However, these everyday choices take on an importance and significance due to the mothers' heightened awareness of the fragility of life, emphasised by our natality. Choices become urgent, they become matters of life and death. These two elements are also brought together when the mother is at her most vulnerable, when she feels unskilled and unconfident. When she does not yet understand, or can make sense of, this new life that she is living. With so much that is new and uncertain, women are faced with continued challenges that continue long after their baby has been born.

Being aware of our choice highlights our freedom—that we are free to choose our lives and the way we live them. We are also free to choose ourselves. The enormity of this choice, and our awareness of our existence, leads to an experience of existential anxiety.

Whilst van Deurzen (2010) suggests there is 'no blueprint for living', similarly there is no one way of being a mother. Every woman is unique and therefore there are as many ways of being a mother as there are women. Each mother's experience will be coloured by their own personal situation, whether this is due to their sexuality, their culture and ethnicity, their social situation or their neurobiological make up. Each will bring with it its own challenges and concerns. However, existential philosophy focuses awareness on the fundamental aspects of our human existence that transcend our individual experiences; the tensions that are caused by being limited in time, and the anxiety and guilt that is experienced through enacting our freedom. An existential approach does not aim to rid us of our anxiety or to make our lives easier or more comfortable. Instead, it contends that by accepting that challenge and difficulty are part of our existential condition, we may be able to find more meaningful ways to live. This is not to diminish the variety of different voices that express the many ways in which women can be mothers, instead it offers a ground from which to view and understand those experiences.

The overarching theme that runs through this book is one of identity and the struggle this creates for women when they become mothers. Identity becomes the fulcrum that brings together the bio-psycho-socio-spiritual dimensions (van Deurzen 2010) of being a mother and demonstrates how interlinked and interconnected these aspects are. Natality, and I would argue maternity too, reveals our embeddedness in the world (Stone 2019). We cannot escape the social context of our lives which has a powerful impact on our sense of ourselves and our identity. This begins in our embodiment and our biology. Our embodiment gives us a sense of identity, which includes a sense of gender and sexuality. But for women embodied identity is still closely bound to their reproductive abilities. This creates a heteronormative ideal of the concept 'woman', which becomes bound to the concept of 'mother'. Coates-Davies notes in Chapter 13, that motherhood is always presented as a binary choice between motherhood or childfreedom, without recognising that for some women motherhood is never a choice to be considered. Body identity is also connected to social norms about what a body should 'do' and how it should 'look'. Women who believe they fall short of these social norms are left with feelings of failure, of their body having let them down and this then connects to their motherhood identity of 'not being good enough'. Yet these norms are socially constructed and create images and myths around the ideas of 'natural childbirth' or the 'maternal instinct'. They create unrealistic expectations in women which do not allow for the myriad ways in which women can become or be mothers. If a woman feels her body is not responding in the way that she expects it should then she feels a 'sense of corporeal homelessness' as discussed in Chapter 3.

Mothers not only experience a sense of homelessness in their bodies, but motherhood can create a sense of not feeling at home in themselves too. Motherhood can be a momentous but confusing time for women. The whole vista of their lives change, but they also become aware of the realities of existence, of uncertainty, and the responsibility and freedom that comes with taking care of a child. The mother's world-view shifts, and she experiences changes in all four dimensions of her life. This evokes a sense of not understanding what is happening—the mother's sense of self changes and yet she still feels the same. Part of this confusion stems from having to grapple with the new social norms that surround the motherhood identity. Mothers often struggle to reconcile their actual experience with the expectations concerning the societal roles they have taken on.

Whilst there have been many advances in equality for women over the years this has only served to create impossible gender norms for mothers to aspire to. Mothers know that they can no longer 'have-it-all' and yet there are still expectations that they must work as if they have no children and mother their children as if they have no work. Witt (2020) observed that society is constructed on the basis of a series of gendered norms and mothers need to work out which takes priority and how they should respond in a given situation. This is the social crisis that mothers face and this struggle often creates such an unbearable tension that seems so unreconcilable at times that their mental health suffers.

This raises interesting questions about how power is exerted in predominately pro-natal societies. Brown (2019) argues that social discourse is geared towards reproduction which has the effect of reducing women to their biology and consigning them to the private sphere of society (Rossiter 1988; Arnold-Baker 2019). Yet women are far from powerless, and it is this aspect that is behind the third and fourth wave feminism movements. Third and fourth wave Feminists, such as Walker (1992), argue that women become marginalised or oppressed in society due to the way gendered norms intersect with each other and with existing power structures. This is most keenly felt in motherhood, where mother's voices and experiences have been effectively silenced (Arnold-Baker 2019), in preference to the predominate social discourse. Milli Hill in her book *Give Birth Like a Feminist* (2019) argues that childbirth is a central feminist issue, where women can regain their power and take control of their bodies through their birthing choices. This is also echoed in the BirthStrike movement against climate change where women are taking control of their reproduction in order to enact system change (Arnold-Baker 2021). The mother's power, therefore, lies in recognising what Kristeva states, as the 'mother's genius' (Kristeva 2002: 301), that women undertake the ultimate 'Creative act' (ibid., 366) that of creating new human beings. It may be difficult for women to know how to harness this maternal power, particularly as new mothers, who feel *thrown* into their new experiences. But in time they can challenge the gendered norms that exist in society, by finding their own way of being a mother based on their own experiences rather than feeling they have to take on an idealised socially constructed version of 'mother'. This book aims to contribute to the much needed change in social discourse around motherhood and whilst it does not capture motherhood in all its diversity it does give voice to a variety of motherhood experiences which show the reality of life for mothers.

Whilst mothers are embedded in a particular social context, this context does not need to determine their identity. As has been shown throughout this book, identity is something that evolves over time, as a process of becoming. The maternal identity is not something that is bestowed onto a woman straight after childbirth, but it emerges out of the mother's experiences and is refined by how she makes sense of her life. In fact Chapter 10 demonstrates how the personal can also influence the social, as Ofori elucidates how first-generation Ghanaian mothers blended their different cultural identities to create a new emerged identity that was unique to each, but which also created a new sense of culture for these mothers.

The social crisis of motherhood emerges from the intersection between the personal and the social, between the private and the public. But it also forms part of the broader existential crisis that mothers experience where they are connected with the fundamentals of human existence. Tillich (1952) noted that existential courage was needed in order to create a life for ourselves despite the limitations that we face, primarily that we are limited in life. Reflecting on our finitude also brings the absurdity of life (Camus 1955) to the fore. Tillich states that we need the 'courage to be' in order to create a sense of ourselves despite the threat of our non-existence. Motherhood highlights those ontological aspects of existence, but this heightened awareness comes at a time of vulnerability for women, where they feel they lack the necessary skills and resources to take on the huge burden of responsibility that they face.

It is no wonder then that mothers can experience difficulties as a response to the enormous changes in their lives, whilst at the same time being bought face to face with the nature of their existence. This may manifest itself in depression or anxiety, or they may feel traumatised or out of control. These can be seen as understandable responses to a challenging situation. It seems, therefore, that motherhood needs a refocus of perspective, to allow for the reality of the mothers' experience. That it can be a joyful, wonderful and longed for experience but at the same time can be difficult, traumatic and overwhelming. When we refocus the motherhood experience as an existential crisis, it begins to make sense for women. They begin to understand the enormity of what has happened to them and it allows them to feel more in control and in touch with their own experience.

An existential perspective on motherhood does not seek to pathologise these experiences but rather to enable mothers to gain a deeper understanding of their lives. Through facing and acknowledging the difficulties that they encounter, women will be able to make better choices for themselves, their children and their family. Through embracing uncertainty, not understanding and not knowing, mothers can find flexibility and new ways of coping with their situation. By seeing the bigger picture mothers begin to understand their own place in it and start to have confidence in finding their own way as a mother.

As the chapters in this book have shown the experience of motherhood fundamentally changes a woman. However, living through difficulty and facing adversity, enables mothers to be transformed in a spiritual sense, to find a more meaningful way of living. Facing up to the prospect of their own death and that of their child's can lead to a more resolute way of living (Heidegger 1962; Arnold-Baker 2015), where mothers are able to make more authentic choices in the way that they live. To find the courage to trust their own experience and to strike out on their own motherhood path, which may feel difficult if it is against the norms of the society in which they live. As with everything in life, the things that we struggle with the most are often the most meaningful for us. Enabling women to see motherhood as an existential re-birth will allow them to take authorship of their lives again rather than feeling at the mercy of circumstance. Through this process, mothers will be able to find ways in which they can enact their power rather than feeling powerless. Motherhood highlights the paradoxical nature of human existence, that life is not a simple case of choosing one thing over another, but it involves a rich tapestry of interconnected elements. Recognising this will enable mothers to have the courage to find a way to be themselves. As after all motherhood is first and foremost a relationship, a relationship that mothers have with themselves, with their babies, other people and with the wider world around them. If we consider motherhood as a relationship rather than a fixed identity, it has the effect of disconnecting societal norms from a sense of self. Relationships are fluid, they change, they are co-created and as has been shown throughout this book so is our sense of identity. If mothers are able to move away from thinking of maternity as an instinct and mothering as a 'natural' part of being a woman, then we can turn towards an idea that motherhood is a relationship that is co-created and emerges out of our experiences. This would allow for the possibility that there is no one way to be a mother and that it is something that each mother creates for herself. As with any relationship, motherhood is something that needs to be worked out and one that evolves over time. Taking this view of motherhood allows women to enact their freedom to choose their own way of expressing that aspect of themselves. This indeed takes courage, existential courage which Arendt notes is 'already present in a willingness to act and speak at all, to insert one's self into the world and begin a story of one's own' (Arendt 2008: 186). This is the heroic task that women face when they become mothers, when their lives and selves have been deconstructed, and they have to begin a new story of their own.

References

Arendt, H. (2008). *The Human Condition.* Chicago: The University of Chicago Press.

Arnold-Baker, C. (2015). *How Becoming a Mother Involves a Confrontation with Existence: An Existential-Phenomenological Exploration of the Experience of*

Early Motherhood. Doctoral thesis Middlesex University and New School of Psychotherapy and Counselling. http://eprints.mdx.ac.uk/18278/.

Arnold-Baker, C. (2019, Spring). The Public-Private Paradox: An Existential Exploration of Mothers in Society. *Self & Society, 47*(1), 7–13.

Arnold-Baker, C. (2021). Birth Strike: Holding the Tension Between Existence and Non-existence. In D. Vakoch & S. Mickey (Eds.), *Eco-Anxiety and Planetary Hope: Confronting Pandemics and the Climate Crisis*. Lanham: Rowman & Littlefield.

Brown, J. (2019). *Birth Strike: The Hidden Fight over Women's Work*. Michigan: PM Press.

Camus, A. (1955 [1942]). *The Myth of Sisyphus*. Trans. J. O'Brian. London: Penguin Books Ltd.

Heidegger, M. (1962 [1927]). *Being and Time*. Trans. J. Macquarrie & E. S. Robinson. Malden, MA and Oxford: Blackwell.

Hill, M. (2019). *Give Birth Like a Feminist: Your Body. Your Baby. Your Choices.* Croydon: CPI Group.

Kristeva, J. (2002). Maternity, Feminism and Female Sexuality. In K. Oliver (Ed.), *The Portable Kristeva*. New York: Columbia University Press.

Rossiter, A. (1988). *From Private to Public: A Feminist Exploration of Early Mothering*. Toronto: The Women's Press.

Stone, A. (2019). *Being Born: Birth and Philosophy*. Oxford: Oxford University Press.

Tillich, P. (1952). *The Courage to Be*. New Haven, CT: Yale University Press.

van Deurzen, E. (2010). *Everyday Mysteries, a Handbook of Existential Psychotherapy* (2nd ed.). Hove, East Sussex: Routledge.

Walker, R. (1992, January). Becoming the Third Wave. *MS*, pp. 39–41.

Witt, C. (2020). Gender Essences. https://aeon.co/essays/would-you-be-the-same-person-if-you-were-a-different-gender (accessed June 2020).

Index

C. Arnold-Baker (ed.), *The Existential Crisis of Motherhood*,
https://doi.org/10.1007/978-3-030-56499-5

www.ingramcontent.com/pod-product-compliance
Lightning Source LLC
Chambersburg PA
CBHW072146010426
42187CB00065B/340
* 9 7 8 3 0 3 0 5 6 4 9 8 8 *